T0358926

The Female Athlete

Editor

SIOBHAN M. STATUTA

CLINICS IN
SPORTS MEDICINE

www.sportsmed.theclinics.com

Consulting Editor
MARK D. MILLER

October 2017 • Volume 36 • Number 4

ELSEVIER

1600 John F. Kennedy Boulevard • Suite 1800 • Philadelphia, Pennsylvania, 19103-2899

http://www.theclinics.com

CLINICS IN SPORTS MEDICINE Volume 36, Number 4
October 2017 ISSN 0278-5919, ISBN-13: 978-0-323-54688-1

Editor: Lauren Boyle
Developmental Editor: Donald Mumford

© **2017 Elsevier Inc. All rights reserved.**

This periodical and the individual contributions contained in it are protected under copyright by Elsevier, and the following terms and conditions apply to their use:

Photocopying

Single photocopies of single articles may be made for personal use as allowed by national copyright laws. Permission of the Publisher and payment of a fee is required for all other photocopying, including multiple or systematic copying, copying for advertising or promotional purposes, resale, and all forms of document delivery. Special rates are available for educational institutions that wish to make photocopies for non-profit educational classroom use. For information on how to seek permission visit www.elsevier.com/permissions or call: (+44) 1865 843830 (UK)/(+1) 215 239 3804 (USA).

Derivative Works

Subscribers may reproduce tables of contents or prepare lists of articles including abstracts for internal circulation within their institutions. Permission of the Publisher is required for resale or distribution outside the institution. Permission of the Publisher is required for all other derivative works, including compilations and translations (please consult www.elsevier.com/permissions).

Electronic Storage or Usage

Permission of the Publisher is required to store or use electronically any material contained in this periodical, including any article or part of an article (please consult www.elsevier.com/permissions). Except as outlined above, no part of this publication may be reproduced, stored in a retrieval system or transmitted in any form or by any means, electronic, mechanical, photocopying, recording or otherwise, without prior written permission of the Publisher.

Notice

No responsibility is assumed by the Publisher for any injury and/or damage to persons or property as a matter of products liability, negligence or otherwise, or from any use or operation of any methods, products, instructions or ideas contained in the material herein. Because of rapid advances in the medical sciences, in particular, independent verification of diagnoses and drug dosages should be made.

Although all advertising material is expected to conform to ethical (medical) standards, inclusion in this publication does not constitute a guarantee or endorsement of the quality or value of such product or of the claims made of it by its manufacturer.

Clinics in Sports Medicine (ISSN 0278-5919) is published quarterly by Elsevier Inc., 360 Park Avenue South, New York, NY 10010-1710. Months of issue are January, April, July, and October. Business and Editorial Offices: 1600 John F. Kennedy Blvd., Ste. 1800, Philadelphia, PA 19103-2899. Customer Service Office: 3251 Riverport Lane, Maryland Heights, MO 63043. Periodicals postage paid at New York, NY and additional mailing offices. Subscription prices are $343.00 per year (US individuals), $627.00 per year (US institutions), $100.00 per year (US students), $389.00 per year (Canadian individuals), $774.00 per year (Canadian institutions), $235.00 (Canadian students), $475.00 per year (foreign individuals), $774.00 per year (foreign institutions), and $235.00 per year (foreign students). Foreign air speed delivery is included in all *Clinics* subscription prices. All prices are subject to change without notice. **POSTMASTER:** Send address changes to *Clinics in Sports Medicine*, Elsevier Health Sciences Division, Subscription Customer Service, 3251 Riverport Lane, Maryland Heights, MO 63043. Customer Service (orders, claims, online, change of address): Elsevier Health Sciences Division, Subscription Customer Service, 3251 Riverport Lane, Maryland Heights, MO 63043. **Tel: 1-800-654-2452 (U.S. and Canada); 314-447-8871 (outside U.S. and Canada). Fax: 314-447-8029. E-mail: journalscustomerservice-usa@elsevier.com (for print support); journalsonlinesupport-usa@ elsevier.com (for online support).**

Reprints. For copies of 100 or more of articles in this publication, please contact the Commercial Reprints Department, Elsevier Inc., 360 Park Avenue South, New York, NY 10010-1710. Tel.: 212-633-3874; Fax: 212-633-3820; E-mail: reprints@elsevier.com.

Clinics in Sports Medicine is covered in *MEDLINE/PubMed (Index Medicus) Current Contents/Clinical Medicine, Excerpta Medica,* and *ISI/Biomed.*

Contributors

CONSULTING EDITOR

MARK D. MILLER, MD
S. Ward Casscells Professor, Head, Division of Sports Medicine, Department of Orthopaedic Surgery, University of Virginia, Charlottesville, Virginia; Team Physician, James Madison University, Director, Miller Review Course, Harrisonburg, Virginia

EDITOR

SIOBHAN M. STATUTA, MD, CAQSM
Director, Primary Care Sports Medicine Fellowship, Associate Professor, Departments of Family Medicine and Physical Medicine and Rehabilitation, Team Physician, University of Virginia Sports Medicine, University of Virginia Health System, Charlottesville, Virginia

AUTHORS

ASHLEY AUSTIN, MD
Department of Family Medicine, University of Virginia Health System, Charlottesville, Virginia

ROBERT W. BATTLE, MD
Professor of Medicine and Pediatrics, Team Cardiologist, Division of Pediatric Cardiology, University of Virginia Health System, University of Virginia, Charlottesville, Virginia

DONNA K. BROSHEK, PhD
John Edward Fowler Professor, Department of Psychiatry and Neurobehavioral Sciences, University of Virginia School of Medicine, Charlottesville, Virginia

JEREMY M. BURNHAM, MD
Sports Medicine and Orthopaedic Surgeon, University of Pittsburgh Medical Center for Sports Medicine, Pittsburgh, Pennsylvania; Sports Medicine at Bone & Joint Clinic, Baton Rouge, Louisiana

BARRY KENT DIDUCH, MD, FAAFP
Primary Care Team Physician, Associate Professor, Department of Sports Medicine, James Madison University, Harrisonburg, Virginia

JAMES E. FERGUSON II, MD, MBA
W. Norman Thornton Jr Professor and Chair, Department of Obstetrics and Gynecology, University of Virginia School of Medicine, Charlottesville, Virginia

JANA M. GOLDBERG, MD
Assistant Professor of Clinical Medicine, Department of Cardiovascular Disease, Hospital of the University of Pennsylvania, Corporal Michael J. Crescenz Department of Veterans Affairs Medical Center, Philadelphia, Pennsylvania

ELIZABETH A. GREGG, PhD
Chair, Associate Professor, Department of Leadership, School Counseling, and Sport Management, University of North Florida, Jacksonville, Florida

VANESSA H. GREGG, MD
Division Director, Obstetrics and Gynecology, Associate Professor, Department of Obstetrics and Gynecology, University of Virginia School of Medicine, University Physicians for Women Northridge, Charlottesville, Virginia

JOHN M. MacKNIGHT, MD, FACSM
Professor, Internal Medicine and Orthopaedic Surgery, Medical Director for Sports Medicine, University of Virginia Health System, University Physicians Charlottesville, Charlottesville, Virginia

AMANDA RACH, PhD
Postdoctoral Fellow, Department of Psychiatry and Neurobehavioral Sciences, University of Virginia School of Medicine, Charlottesville, Virginia

JACOB E. RESCH, PhD
Assistant Professor, Department of Kinesiology, University of Virginia, Charlottesville, Virginia

KELLY A. ROSSI, MS, RD, CSSD
Associate Director of Sports Nutrition, Department of Athletics, University of Virginia, Charlottesville, Virginia

SIOBHAN M. STATUTA, MD, CAQSM
Director, Primary Care Sports Medicine Fellowship, Associate Professor, Departments of Family Medicine and Physical Medicine and Rehabilitation, Team Physician, University of Virginia Sports Medicine, University of Virginia Health System, Charlottesville, Virginia

SAMUEL WALTON, MEd
Doctoral Student, Department of Kinesiology, University of Virginia, Charlottesville, Virginia

SHELBY C. WHITE, MD
Fellow, Department of Pediatrics, Division of Pediatric Cardiology, University of Virginia Children's Hospital Heart Center, University of Virginia, Charlottesville, Virginia

NANCY I. WILLIAMS, ScD, FACSM
Noll Laboratory, Department of Kinesiology, Women's Health and Exercise Laboratories, Penn State University, University Park, Pennsylvania

VONDA WRIGHT, MD, MS
Medical Director, University of Pittsburgh Medical Center Lemieux Sports Complex, Cranberry Township, Pennsylvania; Founder, Women's Health Conversations Conference, Director, PRIMA-Performance and Research Initiative for Masters Athletes, Associate Professor, Orthopaedic Surgeon, University of Pittsburgh Medical Center for Sports Medicine, Pittsburgh, Pennsylvania

Contents

Exercise can have significant effects on gastrointestinal diseases. Regular, moderate exercise can impart beneficial effects for the intestinal microbiome, irritable bowel syndrome symptoms, and inflammatory bowel disease. High-intensity training or prolonged endurance training, on the other hand, can have negative effects on these same entities. Female athletes report a higher prevalence of irritable bowel syndrome and celiac disease, and furthermore, have gastrointestinal symptoms modulated by the menstrual cycle. Management of gastrointestinal problems in the athletic population is widespread and includes training adjustments, dietary measures, and medicine management of symptoms.

Despite more than 3 decades of research on the Female Athlete Triad, research gaps remain. Although low energy availability (EA) is the key etiologic factor in the Triad and the pathways to low EA are varied, its effects can be modified by several factors. Accurate screening, diagnosis, and treatment of disordered eating are a challenge; however, recent techniques combined with novel educational and behavior interventions prove promising. Recently published practice-based guidelines have helped to translate Triad science and should improve as they are refined. This article identifies the current state of research and distinguishes areas that require further investigation.

Disorders of bone density are especially prevalent among athletic women. The severity of bone loss ranges from osteopenia to frank osteoporosis. In female athletes, a higher incidence of osteoporosis is due to a decreased rate of bone accretion in youth, often as a result of hormonal deficiency and/or excessive exercise. Low bone mass poses a particular challenge for athletes because it predisposes to stress-related bone injuries and increases the risk of osteoporosis and insufficiency fractures with aging. This article reviews the pathophysiology of bone thinning in premenopausal and postmenopausal women, the impact of exercise, and the treatment options presently available.

As female athlete sports participation has continued to increase, the rate of anterior cruciate ligament (ACL) rupture in female athletes has also increased. Individualized, patient-specific treatment is crucial to achieving optimal outcomes; ACL reconstruction must accurately restore native ACL anatomy and address any concomitant injury to secondary stabilizers. Rehabilitation programs should target hip, core, and trunk neuromuscular control; allow adequate time for graft ligamentization; and address the psychosocial needs of the athlete.

Sport concussion (SC) has emerged as a major health concern in the medical community and general public owing to increased research and media attention, which has primarily focused on male athletes. Female athletes have an equal, if not increased, susceptibility to SC. An ever-growing body of research continues to compare male and female athletes in terms of SC before and after an injury. Clinicians must be cognizant of this literature to make evidence-based clinical decisions when providing care to female athletes and discern between dated and/or unsupported claims in terms of SC.

Routine exercise should be recommended to healthy pregnant women after consultation with an obstetric provider. Even pregnant women who have not been exercising regularly can gradually increase their exercise during pregnancy. Regular exercise during pregnancy promotes overall wellness and helps maintain appropriate gestational weight gain and appropriate fetal weight gain. Exercise in pregnancy may also reduce hypertensive disorders of pregnancy and gestational diabetes and may be associated with shorter first stage of labor and decreased risk for cesarean section. Exercise in pregnancy is safe for pregnant women and their fetuses and can have multiple health benefits.

The Female Athlete
CLINICS IN SPORTS MEDICINE

RELATED INTEREST

Orthopedic Clinics of North America, July 2017 (Vol. 48, Issue 3)
Orthobiologics
Frederick M. Azar, *Editor*
Available at: http://www.orthopedic.theclinics.com/

THE CLINICS ARE AVAILABLE ONLINE!
Access your subscription at:
www.theclinics.com

Foreword

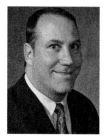

Mark D. Miller, MD
Consulting Editor

As sports medicine physicians, our knowledge and expertise regarding the specific treatment of female athletes continue to grow as research, clinical experiences, and surgical outcomes guide our progress. Title IX, certainly not universally well received by many traditional college athletic departments, has now been in place for 45 years and has played a major role toward leveling the playing field with respect to all aspects of women's athletics. Our gratitude extends both to women athletes and to colleagues who have led the charge to address issues and challenges associated with the specific care of female athletes. This issue of *Clinics in Sports Medicine*, both timely and necessary, offers our best thinking on a variety of topics. My sincere appreciation to Dr Siobhan Statuta, an excellent primary care sports medicine specialist at our institution, for putting together this important issue.

Comprehensive coverage of a topic is best initiated with an understanding of history, and this issue is no exception. This is followed with articles addressing specific issues that are of importance to the female athlete and to those of us who take care of them. This includes comprehensive reviews of cardiovascular considerations, nutrition, gastrointestinal conditions, the female athlete triad, bony disorders, the ACL (a topic well recognized by orthopedic sports medicine physicians), concussion, and pregnancy. In sum, this is an excellent update and review of important issues concerning the female athlete. Congratulations and sincere thanks, Dr Statuta!

Mark D. Miller, MD
S. Ward Casscells Professor
Division of Sports Medicine
Department of Orthopaedic Surgery
University of Virginia
400 Ray C. Hunt Drive, Suite 330
Charlottesville, VA 22908-0159, USA

E-mail address:
mdm3p@virginia.edu

Clin Sports Med 36 (2017) ix
http://dx.doi.org/10.1016/j.csm.2017.07.015
0278-5919/17/© 2017 Published by Elsevier Inc.

sportsmed.theclinics.com

Preface

The Female Athlete

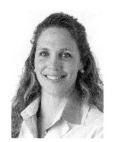

Siobhan M. Statuta, MD, CAQSM
Editor

Women's participation in sport has risen in the last 50 years, and boy, is that an understatement! (pun intended). This is fact, regardless of the level of sport. Consider the marathon of all marathons: Boston. It doesn't matter whether you credit Bobbi Gibb for being the first female finisher of this race in 1966 when she snuck in unofficially without a number, or you recognize Kathrine Switzer who successfully completed the race the following year as a bibbed runner due to a registration error. *Both* are considered pioneers and were retroactively acknowledged as race champions by the Boston Athletic Association years later. It was finally in 1971 that women were officially permitted to register and run the race. Over the years, the number of female finishers has skyrocketed to an astounding 45% of registered runners: 13,698 in 2017![1] Stories like this are not unique to the running community alone, but are evidenced across sport and level of competition as well. In 1970, there were approximately 16,000 female intercollegiate athletes. By 2016, this number exceeded 214,000![2] In the high school arena, the 2016 National Survey reported girls' athletic participation had reached an all-time high: over 3,324,000. Moreover, this was the 27th consecutive year of increased sport participation by girls in high school.[3] Girls recreational sports at even younger ages are established as well. Girls have greater access to a wider array of sports and are getting involved at younger ages, and the rise in participant numbers proves this.

Parallel to this upsurge in female athletics, the subspecialty of sports medicine has also evolved. With it now comes the unique challenge of treating these female athletes. Female athletes, though able to play and maneuver similarly to their male counterparts, are indeed different beings. Anatomical and physiological variances place women in a separate category than men, oftentimes placing them at greater risk for injury. It is imperative that the sports medicine clinician be aware of the nuances of the female athlete. By recognizing these distinctions, it allows the sports medicine physician the ability to better counsel the female athlete on nutrition, psychology, physical

Clin Sports Med 36 (2017) xi–xii
http://dx.doi.org/10.1016/j.csm.2017.07.014
0278-5919/17/© 2017 Published by Elsevier Inc.

sportsmed.theclinics.com

conditioning, the prevention of injuries, and increasing performance. It is our duty, as the medical team, to stay current with the latest evidence, in order to more successfully serve as educator and care provider. This female-focused issue of *Clinics in Sports Medicine* provides a variety of challenging and dynamic topics with the aim not only to provide a comprehensive review but also to serve as a reference for years to come.

A special thank you to all the contributing authors who took time out of their busy lives to research, create, and contribute such valuable articles to this issue. It has been a true honor to collaborate on this project. Finally, I'd like to especially thank Dr Mark Miller for his mentoring and support throughout the years as well as for providing me this platform to further the knowledge and education of fellow clinicians and professionals alike. Enjoy!

Siobhan M. Statuta, MD, CAQSM
Department of Family Medicine
University of Virginia Health System
PO Box 800729
Charlottesville, VA 22908-0729, USA

E-mail address:
SMS5BB@virginia.edu

REFERENCES

1. Boston Athletic Association. 2017 Boston marathon statistics. Available at: http://registration.baa.org/2017/cf/Public/iframe_Statistics.htm. Accessed April 28, 2017.
2. 2015-16 NCAA sports sponsorship and participation rates report. Available at: http://www.ncaapublications.com/productdownloads/PR1516.pdf. Accessed April 28, 2017.
3. 2015-16 High school athletics participation survey. The National Federation of State High School Associations. Available at: http://www.nfhs.org/ParticipationStatistics/PDF/2015-16_Sports_Participation_Survey.pdf. Accessed April 28, 2017.

Women in Sport
Historical Perspectives

Elizabeth A. Gregg, PhD[a],*, Vanessa H. Gregg, MD[b]

KEYWORDS

- Title IX • Women in sport • History of women in sport

KEY POINTS

- Historically, sport has been a male-dominated realm. Women were initially discouraged from participating in exercise and sport activities because they were thought to be too fragile.
- Over the course of the twentieth century, women have gained greater access to athletic participation opportunities. This access is largely attributable to Title IX of the Educational Amendments of 1972.
- Although women have not been granted the same opportunities to participate in professional sport than men, there are still examples of professional sport leagues for women with long and storied histories.

INTRODUCTION

Much like other facets of society, the current state of women in sport is the result of a long and varied history. In the United States, Victorian ideals shaped not only appropriate behavior for men and women in domestic life but also in professional work and, ultimately, in sport participation. Medical experts during the nineteenth century believed that the female body was too fragile to handle social stressors, the rigor of intense study, working long hours, or engaging in intense exercise. It was believed that engaging in these types of behaviors could lead to a range of health conditions, including the inability to bear healthy children, and a host of other negative ramifications. Physicians also believed that girls were at risk, particularly those at the age of puberty, of depleting their "vital force" or lifetime energy capacity.[1] Girls who chose to participate in vigorous activity were thought to be at risk of becoming sterile,

Disclosure statement: The author has nothing to disclose.
[a] Department of Leadership, School Counseling, and Sport Management, University of North Florida, 1 UNF Drive, Jacksonville, FL 32224, USA; [b] Department of Obstetrics and Gynecology, University of Virginia School of Medicine, University Physicians for Women Northridge, UVA Medical Park Northridge, Third Floor, 2955 Ivy Road, (250 West), Charlottesville, VA 22903, USA
* Corresponding author.
E-mail address: liz.gregg@unf.edu

weak, or masculine. The growth of competitive sport for girls and women was restricted by these medical fallacies.[1]

The Victorian ideals described earlier prevented the average woman from taking part in widespread sport participation during the age of modernization of sport in America, which began during the mid-1800s. Although most competitive sports were reserved for men, upper-class women had access to a range of individual sports, such as golf, tennis, archery, and croquet. All of these forms of activities fit the Victorian ideal; participation did not necessitate vigorous activity, and each could be played in sex-appropriate clothing, which consisted of dresses and corsets.[2,3]

As Americans began to understand the benefits gained through sport participation, such as teamwork, communication skills, work ethic, and respect for authority, youth and adult sport programs proliferated nationwide during the late nineteenth century.[3–5] Although young boys and men enjoyed fully competitive activities that created desirable masculine traits, girls and women participated almost exclusively in noncompetitive recreation.[6] Staying with the desirable Victorian ideals, women enjoyed archery, croquet, tennis, sailing, skating, and hiking. Some literature indicates that during the late 1800s, women's colleges across the country allowed additional forms of sport to be played, such as crew, swimming, and golf. At Smith College, women competed in the first collegiate game of basketball in 1892.[7]

THE DEVELOPMENT OF COMPETITIVE SPORT PROGRAMS FOR WOMEN

Throughout the 1890s and into the twentieth century, basketball became one of the most prolific sports for women nationwide. Teams formed across the country, and women's rules designed to decrease vigor and physical contact were created. Growth occurred rapidly after the Young Men's Christian Association (YMCA) published the rules in a newsletter distributed nationwide.[3] The rapid growth alarmed some female leaders of physical education programs, which provided structure, support, and coaching for girls' sport programs. At the same time, society witnessed a great change in 1920 when the Equal Suffrage Amendment passed, which allowed women more social freedom and access to employment.[8] This era was considered a golden age for women, as more freedom in dress allowed for enhanced athletic participation. Perhaps one of the most memorable figures to appear in the popular press during this era was the Gibson Girl. Akin to the flappers of the roaring twenties, the Gibson Girl was an athletic-looking woman dressed in sporting attire who frequently appeared in women's magazines and other publications.[7]

Because of the concerns related to girls participating in competitive sports on a broad scale, many female leaders thought that a governing body for women's athletics was necessary to ensure the health and well-being of female athletes. One such group that emerged was the National Amateur Athletic Federation (NAAF).[9] The NAAF had beliefs that aligned with opponents of women's athletics. Based on unfounded medical beliefs, the NAAF and critics of women's sport believed intense physical activity could lead to masculine behavior, endanger the reproductive health of female participants, and cause anxiety. NAAF leaders were also troubled by the prospect that women's intercollegiate athletic programs would adopt a model that emphasized entertainment, professionalism, and commercialization similar to the men's model of the era, which critics stated were variables that distracted student-athletes from their studies. The NAAF evolved into the Division of Girls and Women in Sport, which later became the Association for Intercollegiate Athletics for Women.[9]

The medical myths that stated intense physical activity and competition were dangerous to women's health were accepted by most female physical educators who controlled school-based sports. These female leaders, believing they were acting in the best interest of their students, moved to alter the manner in which athletic programs were structured on college campuses. In most cases, highly competitive athletics for female students were virtually eliminated from institutions of higher learning. Noncompetitive athletics were encouraged, and Play Days became the norm.[10] Play Days were noncompetitive sport days for women held on college campuses nationwide; their slogan, "a sport for every girl and every girl in a sport,"[11] highlighted the recreational nature of the events.

For nearly 40 years, the only forms of athletic competition available to girls and women were non–school-based sport programs and intramural-type events. During the feminist movement of the 1960s, sport was one vehicle feminist leaders used to lobby for greater equality for women. With the help of leaders, such as Billy Jean King and the National Organization of Women, sport offerings for women expanded on college campuses and in society in general. There were also 3 pieces of legislation passed during the period from 1960 to 1980 that created legal pathways to expand opportunities for women. Although not written exclusively for the purposes of sport, the reach of each extended to women's sport.[11] The Civil Rights Act of 1964, the use of the 14th Amendment to the Constitution in judicial lawsuits (1973), and Title IX of the Education Amendments Act (1972) were all significant in creating opportunities for women in various facets of society.[11,12]

TITLE IX OF THE EDUCATION AMENDMENTS ACT

The most significant law for women's athletics was Title IX of the Education Amendments Act, which passed in 1972. Title IX explicitly states "No person in the United States shall, on the basis of sex, be excluded from participation in, be denied the benefits of, or be subjected to discrimination under, any educational program or activity receiving Federal financial assistance."[13] Title IX consists of 3 separate, yet interrelated parts. All federally funded institutions must prove their compliance with one or more areas of Title IX.

Part I of Title IX addresses overall equivalence, which includes athletic scholarship dollars offered to men and women. The provisions of equivalent areas are covered under Part II. All educational institutions are required to allocate women's athletic programs with the same benefits, opportunities, and treatment that their men's athletic programs receive. The Title IX Compliance Investigators Manual outlines 12 areas assessed to determine if an institution is compliant. Examples of assessed areas include (but are not limited to) the allocation of equipment and supplies, provisions of locker rooms and support services, and compensation of coaches and tutors. Part III of Title IX addresses the accommodation of student interests and abilities "to the extent necessary to provide equal opportunity in the selection of sports and levels of competition available to both sexes."[13] Every educational program receiving federal financial assistance is required to abide by the mandates outlined in Title IX. A lack of compliance could potentially lead to a loss of federal funding.[13]

WOMEN'S INTERCOLLEGIATE ATHLETICS

Just before the passage of Title IX, leaders in women's physical education and athletic programs once again recognized the need for the presence of a national governing body for women's intercollegiate sport. The Association for Intercollegiate Athletics for Women (AIAW) was established in the months preceding the passage of Title IX in 1971.[14] It was the first and only governing body of intercollegiate athletics formed on an educational platform. The organization was committed to keeping academics as the priority for their student athletes. They established a student-centered policy intended to maximize the holistic development of women participating in collegiate athletic teams. The women of the AIAW sought to avoid the "harmful elements of governance" evident in the National Collegiate Athletic Association's (NCAA) governance structure.[15,16] For example, athletic scholarships based on ability were initially prohibited. The minimum grade point average requirement was higher than that required for men. Whereas male athletes were forced to forfeit a year of eligibility on transfer, AIAW transfer students were granted immediate eligibility. The AIAW also refrained from offering per diem allowances to schools participating in postseason tournaments, a factor that would eventually contribute to its demise.[17]

Throughout the expansion of women's intercollegiate athletic programs in America, the NCAA played a significant, yet often controversial role. For example, in 1965 and 1966, the NCAA publicly stated their lack of interest in women's athletics.[16,18] Following a presentation by members of the Division of Girls and Women in Sport at an NCAA convention highlighting the strengths of women's athletic programs at the college level, the NCAA ratified their bylaws to officially state that their postseason tournaments were for male student athletes only. This example is one of many actions and statements by the NCAA that created distrust toward them by female athletic administrators.[10,16]

Although the AIAW's model of governance was seemingly well suited for students interested in participating on varsity athletic teams while pursuing an undergraduate degree, that model did not prove to have staying power. Many scholars attribute the failure of the AIAW to the increase in the NCAA's financial stake in controlling women's intercollegiate athletics. Interestingly, before the NCAA began offering national championships for women's teams, they first attempted to limit their program offerings exclusively to men and even tried to later restrict the scope of Title IX. Senator John Tower, a supporter of the NCAA, proposed the Tower Amendments, which were drafted with the intent to limit the scope of Title IX[19] to only nonrevenue sports. The Tower Amendments were arguably one of the most explicit attempts by the NCAA and its supporters to prevent the development of varsity athletic teams for women.[13]

Locked in heated legal battles with the NCAA for several years, the AIAW exhausted much of their financial resources struggling for control over women's intercollegiate athletics. This high financial burden associated with defending the legal position of the AIAW was documented by Wushanley in 2004.[16] Margot Policy, the attorney responsible for leading the legal charge against the NCAA, became a controversial figure in the history of women's intercollegiate athletics. The tremendous legal fees accrued by the AIAW detracted from the organization's ability to offer high-quality athletic programs to their member institutions. During their peak, the AIAW offered 41 national championships in 19 sports to more than 6000 teams in 960 member colleges and universities.[15] Further, more than 90% of women's programs were coached and administered by women. For all practical purposes, women were successfully leading their intercollegiate athletic programs into a new era; however, those successes within the AIAW were short-lived.[13,17]

Despite the best attempts of the women of the AIAW to remain in control of women's intercollegiate athletic programs, the NCAA began offering Division I national championships for women in 1981. Additionally, the NCAA offered its member institutions the option of adding women's programs without an initiation fee and offered to pay the travel costs of these national championships. Most member schools opted to align their women's programs with the well-established NCAA organization. Crippled financially, the AIAW was without the means to compete with the lucrative offer set forth by the NCAA. After an unsuccessful lawsuit filed by the AIAW charging the NCAA with antitrust violations, the AIAW organization ceased operations in 1982.[16]

Under NCAA control, participation and employment trends in women's intercollegiate athletics changed dramatically. According to Acosta and Carpenter (2014),[20] the total number of athletic participants has almost tripled since the passing of Title IX. During the 2015 to 2016 academic year, there were about 212,000 women competing in NCAA sports, a 25.7% increase over the previous 10 years. The total number of women's teams also increased by 14.2% during this same period.[21] Yet, although participation opportunities have grown tremendously, women who aspire to work in intercollegiate athletic administrations have not fared as well. In 1972 when Title IX passed, more than 90% of women's teams were coached by women. Today, roughly 43% of women's athletic teams have a female head coach.[20] In administration, about 18% of all athletic administrators in NCAA programs are women. More than 90% of women's athletic program administrators were women when Title IX passed into law in 1972. Currently, about 83% of all athletic directors are men.[20,22]

WOMEN IN PROFESSIONAL SPORT

Despite the fact that sport was viewed as an activity for boys and men during the late nineteenth and early twentieth centuries, sport participation grew rapidly in America.[3] In New York City and surrounding regions, sport developed from merely a pastime into a modernized, formalized enterprise used for entertaining the masses.[23] Sporting fraternities were one social group that helped modernize sport in the city. Perhaps the most significant sporting fraternity was the New York Knickerbockers Baseball Club. Established in 1845 by Alexander Cartwright and a group of business people, the Knickerbockers set the rules of baseball and popularized the sport in the city. Thanks to technological advancements, such as the printing press, modern railroad, telegraph, and other improvements, sport rapidly spread nationwide. Recognizing the potential profitability of baseball, William H. Cammeyer was the first to build a fence around a baseball field and charge admission in 1862.[24] Cammeyer kicked off what is now known as the enclosure movement, which was essentially the beginning of the commercial model of team sports, and America's love affair with baseball.[24,25]

Baseball was a sport that women were able to enjoy during the early half of the twentieth century. When World War II broke out and professional baseball seemed to be at risk, chewing gum magnet and sport entrepreneur Phillip K. Wrigley recognized an opportunity. Although softball was the most popular sport for women in 1943, Wrigley believed women could play a version of this men's game. He established the All-American Girls Professional Baseball League (AAGPBL) in 1943 to fill the void in entertainment created by the war.[24,26] Originally, the league consisted of 4 teams located in the Midwest; the AAGPBL played 108 games in front of more than 176,000 fans during the league's first season in 1943.

Popularized by the film *A League of Their Own,* Wrigley ensured that AAGPBL strictly adhered to Victorian ideals. League participants were required to wear short skirts, and the players were required to attend a charm school conducted by Helena Rubenstein's famed Chicago-based beauty salon and finishing school.[25] Women were coached on how to display a feminine image, apply makeup, and learn proper manners.[27,28] The model was successful; the league grew to 10 teams during the 1950s. At the height of the AAGPL's popularity, the league attracted nearly 1 million fans a year.[25] Despite its initial successes, the league could not sustain itself long-term. Because of declining attendance, the league folded in 1954.

The Ladies Professional Golf Association (LPGA) is the longest-running professional sport organization for women in America.[29,30] Founded in 1943 as the Women's Professional Golf Association, the tour evolved into the LPGA in 1949.[29] Much like Wrigley had done with the sport of baseball in the late nineteenth century, sport promoter Fred Corcoran recognized a potential lucrative business opportunity by running a women's golf circuit. Unlike the men's professional golf tour, the LPGA was managed primarily by tour players. In 1950, the tour had a total purse of about $50,000 for 14 events.[30,31]

During the 1960s and 1970s, the LPGA secured its first title sponsor and television agreement for the Women's US Open. Under the direction of LPGA Commissioner Ray Volpe (former vice president of the National Hockey League), the tour undertook an organizational restructuring in the late 1970s. The player-controlled executive board established under the direction of Corcoran was dissolved, and a board of directors consisting of nonplaying members was created. Volpe was also proved to be a creative marketer who understood that by using the sex appeal of tour players, he could attract larger crowds. Through his skillful use of the media, Volpe grew corporate sponsorship by 40% in 3 years.[30,31] Over the course of his tenure, the LPGA experienced its most profitable years. Volpe remained commissioner until 2005.

Carolyn Vesper Bivens assumed control of a healthy organization when she became the commissioner of the LPGA. During Bivens' tenure, there were several missteps, including requiring tour speakers to speak English to the media as well as decisions regarding tournament locations. Bivens stepped down in July of 2009[32] at which point the LPGA's current commissioner, Michael Whan, took over in 2010.

Under Whan's leadership, the LPGA has regained market share lost during the Bivens' administration. The LPGA, the oldest professional sport organization for women, currently hosts 35 events and offered a record high $67 million in prize money during the 2016 season. Television ratings are also up by 40% in 2016.[33] Despite a period of uncertainty, the LPGA is poised for continued success.

BENEFITS OF SPORT PARTICIPATION FOR WOMEN

Girls and women are benefitting from sport participation in a variety of ways. Scholars have determined that high school girls who participate in interscholastic sport are likely to get better grades and are less likely to have unintended pregnancies.[34,35] Women and girls who play sports regularly have higher levels of self-confidence and self-esteem and lower levels of depression. Collegiate athletes also fare well after their eligibility has expired. For example, it has been determined that former intercollegiate female athletes are more likely to be employed full-time after graduation. Former female athletes not only outperform female nonathletes but also their male peers. When it comes to overall health, former intercollegiate athletes are 14% more likely to thrive in terms of overall physical well-being.[13,21,36]

SUMMARY

Much like other facets of society, sport was shaped by Victorian ideals that positioned women in the home. Proper forms of exercise for women during the nineteenth century were nonvigorous activities that could be completed in appropriate feminine attire.[2,3] During the twentieth century, sport solidified its position as a vastly popular form of entertainment. Because the 1920s was a liberal era in America, women gained opportunities to compete in sport on a wider scale. Participation opportunities for women grew exponentially when Title IX of the Education Amendments became law in 1972.[12,13] Although there was some initial confusion regarding the scope of Title IX, it was clear that the landmark law would have lasting effects on opportunities for girls and women to compete in sport. After the NCAA assumed control of women's inter-collegiate athletics in 1981, programs expanded nationally.[13,36] Women have achieved many successes in professional competition across a variety of sports. Overall, women are well positioned to continue their ascent in sport. Although true sex equity has yet to be realized, there are countless examples of success in the development of women's sport; that trajectory will likely continue to be upward.

REFERENCES

1. Smith-Rosenberg C, Rosenberg C. The female animal: medical and biological views of woman and her role in nineteenth-century America. J Am Hist 1973; 60(2):332–56.
2. Adelman M. A sporting time: New York City and the rise of modern athletics, 1820–70. Urbana (IL): University of Illinois Press; 1986.
3. Vertinsky PA. The eternally wounded woman: women, doctors, and exercise in the late nineteenth century. Manchester (United Kingdom): Manchester University Press; 1990.
4. Fraser-Thomas J, Côté J, Deakin J. Youth sport programs: an avenue to foster positive youth development. Phys Education Sport Pedagogy 2005;10(1):19–40.
5. Wiersma L. Risks and benefits of youth sport specialization: perspectives and recommendations. Pediatr Exerc Sci 2000;12(1):13–22.
6. Messner M. Sports and male domination: the female athlete as contested ideological terrain. Sociol Sport J 1988;5(3):197–211.
7. Hult J, Trekell M. A century of women's basketball. From frailty to final four. Reston (VA): AAHPERD Publications Sales; 1991.
8. DuBois E. Working women, class relations, and suffrage militance: Harriot Stanton Blatch and the New York woman suffrage movement, 1894-1909. J Am Hist 1987;74(1):34–58.
9. Theriot N. Towards a new sporting ideal: the Women's Division of the National Amateur Athletic Federation. Frontiers 1978;3(1):1–7.
10. Hooker JH. A history of the women's sports program at Memphis State University [dissertation]. Mississippi: University of Mississippi; 1988.
11. Hult J. Women's struggle for governance in US amateur athletics. Int Rev Sociol Sport 1989;24(3):249–63.
12. Lopiano D. Modern history of women in sports: twenty-five years of Title IX. Clin Sports Med 2000;19(2):163–73.
13. Carpenter L, Acosta R. Title IX. Champaign (IL): Human Kinetics; 2005.
14. Hutchcraft K. Association for intercollegiate athletics for women. J Phys Educ Recreation Dance 1976;47(9):30–1.
15. Hult J. NAGWS and AIAW: the strange and wondrous journey to the athletic summit, 1950–1990. J Phys Educ Recreation Dance 1999;70(4):24–31.
16. Wushanley Y. Playing nice and losing: the struggle for control of women's intercollegiate athletics, 1960-2000. Syracuse (NY): Syracuse University Press; 2004.
17. Whisenant W, Pedersen P, Obenour B. Success and gender: determining the rate of advancement for intercollegiate athletic directors. Sex Roles 2002;47(9–10): 485–91.
18. Swaton B. Girls can play, too: has the lack of female leadership in NCAA athletics become an afterthought. Seton Hall J Sports Ent L 2010;20(1):2–36.
19. Lovett D, Lowry C. Women and the NCAA: not separate—not equal. J Sport Management 1995;9(3):244–8.

20. Acosta RV, Carpenter LJ. Woman in intercollegiate sport: a longitudinal, national study. Thirty-Seven Year Update, 1977-2014. Available at: www.acostacarpenter. org. Accessed February 1, 2017.

21. Sport sponsorship and participation research. National Collegiate Athletic Association Web site. 2016. Available at: http://www.ncaa.org/about/resources/research/sports-sponsorship-and-participation-research. Accessed February 27, 2017.

22. Smith A, Taylor E, Hardin R. Women and mentoring in collegiate athletics. Mentor Tutor Partnership Learn 2016;24(5):346–64.

23. Booth D. The field: truth and fiction in sport history. United Kingdom: Taylor & Francis; 2005.

24. Rader B. American sports: from the age of folk games to the age of televised sports. 6th edition. United Kingdom: Routledge; 2008.

25. Rader B, editor. Early innings: a documentary history of baseball. Lincoln (NE): University of Nebraska Press; 1997. p. 1825–908.

26. Pedersen PM, Thibault L, editors. Contemporary sport management. 5th edition. Champaign (IL): Human Kinetics; 2014.

27. Fidler M. The origins and history of the All-American Girls Professional Baseball League. Jefferson (NC): McFarland Publishing; 2010.

28. Sargent J. We were the All-American Girls: interviews with players of the AAGPBL, 1943-1954. Jefferson (NC): McFarland Publishing; 2013.

29. Kahn L. The LPGA: the unauthorized version: the history of the Ladies Professional Golf Association. Santa Clara (CA): Group Fore Productions; 1996.

30. Rodenberg R, Gregg E, Fielding L. Age eligibility rules in women's professional golf: a legal eagle or an antitrust bogey? J Leg Aspects Sport 2009;19(2):103–20.

31. Crosset T. Outsiders in the clubhouse: the world of women's professional golf. Albany (NY): Suny Press; 1995.

32. Shipnuck A. LPGA Commission Carolyn Bivens was undone by unflinching commitment to her vision for the tour. Tampa (FL): Golf Website; 2009. Available at: http://www.golf.com/tour-and-news/lpga-commissioner-carolyn-bivens-was-undone-unflinching-commitment-her-vision-tour. Accessed February 20, 2017.

33. Shackelford G. Forward press: LPGA commish Mike Whan is seeing the fruits of his efforts. Golf Digest website; 2016. Available at: http://www.golfdigest.com/story/forward-press-lpga-commish-mike-whan-is-seeing-the-fruits-of-his-efforts. Accessed February 20, 2017.

34. Benefits – why sports participation for girls and women. Women's Sports Foundation. Available at: https://www.womenssportsfoundation.org/wp-content/uploads/2016/08/benefits-why-sports-participation-for-girls-and-women-the-foundation-position. pdf. Accessed March 1, 2017.

35. Female student-athletes win big on great jobs, lives. Washington, DC: Gallup; 2016. Available at: http://wwwgallup.com/opinion/gallup/189227/female-student-athletes-win-big-great-jobs-lives.aspx. Accessed March 1, 2017.

36. Gregg E, Fielding L. The implementation of Title IX at Indiana University: a historical case study. J Contemp Sport 2016;10(4):241–55.

Cardiovascular Considerations in the Female Athlete

Shelby C. White, MD[a], Jana M. Goldberg, MD[b],*,
Robert W. Battle, MD[c]

KEYWORDS

- Athlete's heart • Female athlete • Congenital heart disease
- Physiologic adaptation to exercise

KEY POINTS

- Sudden cardiac death (SCD) in athletes is rare and more common in men than women. Earlier studies have cited hypertrophic cardiomyopathy (HCM) as the primary cause of SCD; however, more recent studies challenge this notion suggesting that AN-SCD may be most common.
- Most studies have described differences in cardiac remodeling between male and female athletes. This may be less significant when adjusting for body mass.
- HCM and the presence of a bicuspid aortic valve are more common in male athletes.
- There is no gender predilection in the disease prevalence of Marfan syndrome.
- Maximum oxygen consumption per unit time (Vo_2) is lower in female athletes than in male athletes, though differences may be less notable when adjusting for body composition.

INTRODUCTION

Cardiac care of athletes, from adolescent to masters, has changed tremendously over the last 2 decades. It is now known that the heart adapts both structurally and electrically to the physiologic stresses placed on it through exercise.[1–8] Additionally, recommendations for participation in athletics for those with known cardiovascular conditions continues to evolve.[9–12]

Disclosure Statement: No disclosures.
[a] Division of Pediatric Cardiology, Department of Pediatrics, UVA Children's Hospital Heart Center, University of Virginia, PO Box 800386, Charlottesville, VA 22908, USA; [b] Department of Cardiovascular Disease, Hospital of the University of Pennsylvania, Corporal Michael J. Crescenz Department of Veterans Affairs Medical Center, 3400 Civic Center Boulevard, Philadelphia, PA 19104, USA; [c] Division of Pediatric Cardiology, University of Virginia Health System, University of Virginia, PO Box 800158, Charlottesville, VA 22908-0158, USA
* Corresponding author. Penn Heart and Vascular Center, Perelman Center for Advanced Medicine, East Pavilion, 2nd Floor, 3400 Civic Center Boulevard, Philadelphia, PA 19104.
E-mail address: jana.goldberg@uphs.upenn.edu

Clin Sports Med 36 (2017) 611–625
http://dx.doi.org/10.1016/j.csm.2017.05.008
0278-5919/17/Published by Elsevier Inc.

Particular nuances exist in regard to cardiovascular care of the female athlete compared with the male athlete. This article explains the differences in female athletes, which should aid in understanding physiologic variation, as well as help in making management decisions as they pertain to cardiac issues.

SUDDEN CARDIAC DEATH: EPIDEMIOLOGY AND GENDER DIFFERENCES

Sudden cardiac death (SCD) is most commonly defined as a sudden unexpected death attributable to a cardiac cause. It is also a sudden death in a structurally normal heart with no other viable explanation and a history consistent with cardiac-related demise that occurred within 1 hour of symptom onset or an unwitnessed death occurring within 24 hours of the person having been alive and well.[13] The reported incidence of SCD in the United States has varied based on the baseline population studied and the different techniques used for case identification, such as media reports, national athlete registries, and insurance claims. The largest study of sudden death in young athletes, ages 8 to 39, estimated an overall incidence of SCD in the United States of 0.61 per 100,000 person-years.[14] Other observational studies report an incidence ranging from 1.6 per 100,000 to 1.9 per 100,000.[15,16] In military recruits, the observed rate of nontraumatic sudden death is 13 per 100,000 recruit-years.[17] In all studies, SCD occurs with greater frequency in men compared with women, with 2.6 per 100,000 athlete-years versus 0.8 per 100,000 athlete-years in a population of National Collegiate Athletic Association (NCAA) athletes.

SCD in athletes is rare and more common in men than women.[15–17]

The most common identifiable causes of SCD in the United States are hypertrophic cardiomyopathy (HCM), myocarditis, coronary artery anomalies, and other cardiomyopathies (eg, dilated and arrhythmogenic right ventricular [RV] dysplasia). Until recently, the most common attributable cause of SCD was HCM; however, there is a large proportion of SCD that has since been labeled presumed or autopsy-negative SCD (AN-SCD) due to the inability of conventional autopsies to detect cardiac channelopathies.[14,16–19] Emerging data suggest that AN-SCD may account for most SCD in athletes, as well as in the general population less than 35 years of age. Given this discrepancy, there is a need for high-quality autopsy data and genetic testing in determining the true proportions of structural heart disease accountable for SCD. Data collected from multiple sites worldwide identify HCM as a much less frequent cause of SCD than previously thought, possibly due to the identification of left ventricular (LV) hypertrophy (LVH) from exercise-related remodeling.[18,20,21] All confirmable causes of SCD are more common in men than women. Maron and colleagues[22] identified a 3.5-fold higher rate of HCM in male athletes. Among noncardiovascular causes of sudden death, trauma, suicide, and drug-related deaths have been identified as the most common. Suicide as a cause of sudden death has been shown to be more common in female athletes than in male athletes.

ATHLETIC REMODELING

Forty years ago, the Morganroth Hypothesis was proposed to explain the physiologic changes that the heart undergoes to accommodate for the stress that exercise puts on it. Morganroth and colleagues[1] found that athletes engaging in isotonic exercise (ie, swimming and running) had a greater LV mass and end-diastolic volume. LV wall thickness in this group was no different than nonathletes. The term for this type of remodeling was coined eccentric hypertrophy (**Fig. 1**). However, those engaging in isometric exercise (ie, wrestling) had greater left-ventricular wall thickness without changes in LV end-diastolic volume when compared with nonathletes. This is described as concentric hypertrophy. These variances in remodeling are due to the differences in physiologic stressors on the heart specific to isotonic versus isometric exercises.[1,23] Additionally, several years of data suggest that the hearts of male and female athletes may adapt differently (see **Fig. 1**).

STRUCTURAL DIFFERENCES

Variability in myocardial wall thicknesses exist and depend on factors such as sex; race; and, in particular, the type of activity (endurance vs strength) an athlete participates in. A clinician's role is to correlate what is objectively measured on examination with what is expected for that unique athlete, whether they are primarily a weight-lifter or a cross-country runner.

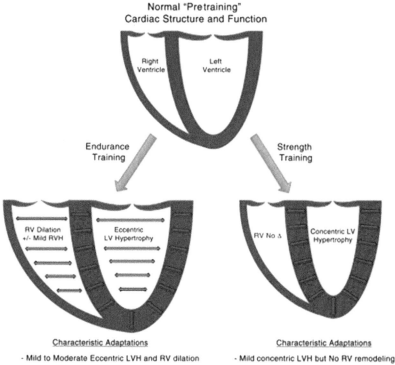

Fig. 1. Cardiac remodeling in endurance versus strength-trained athletes. LVEF, left ventricular ejection fraction. (*From* Weiner RB, Baggish AL. Exercise-induced cardiac remodelling. Prog Cardiovasc Dis 2012;54(5):380–6; with permission.)

Several studies have demonstrated athletic remodeling of the heart in female athletes. Compared with nonathletes, female athletes have greater LV end-diastolic diameter and LV wall thickness by echocardiogram and MRI. Overall, female athletes have smaller absolute dimensions than male athletes[3–6]

In particular, endurance athletics exerts a greater impact on LV cavity dimensions when compared with strength-trained athletes.[3,4] This has been demonstrated both by echocardiogram and cardiac MRI (CMRI). One study examining 600 female Olympians found these athletes displayed larger LV end-diastolic cavity dimensions (mean ± SD) (49 ± 4 mm). LV cavity dimensions exceeded normal limits (>54 mm) in 8%; 1% of these were within the range of dilated cardiomyopathy (≥60 mm). LV cavity size was most affected in those who participated in endurance sports, such as cycling, cross-country skiing, and rowing.[3]

There is an observed increase in RV size in similar sports.[24] RV dilatation, in particular, is found more in endurance rather than strength-trained athletes.[23]

In addition to cavity dilatation, several studies have suggested that female athletes may have increased wall thickness.[3,24–26] By echocardiogram, female athletes have been found to have a greater LV wall thickness than controls (8.2 ± 0.9 mm vs 7.2 ± 0.6 mm; P<.001).[3] By CMRI, a maximum observed reported LV wall thickness was 12 mm.[26] Furthermore, these differences between male and female remodeling-in terms of wall thickness-may be present from adolescence.[8]

Other studies have challenged the notion that the hearts of men and women remodel differently in the setting of athletics. Women tend to have smaller body and chest dimensions, as well as a higher proportion of body fat. When adjusting for lean body mass, recent studies suggest there may not be significant differences between male and female athlete in terms of LV cavity dimensions.[27,28]

In addition to sex differences, race has also been observed to affect athletic remodeling of the heart. Black female athletes demonstrated greater LV wall thickness (9.2 ± 1.2 mm vs 8.6 ± 1.2 mm, P<.001) and LV mass (187.2 ± 42 g vs 172.3 ± 42 g, P = .008) compared with white female athletes.[6] In that particular study, none of the black athletes had LV wall thickness exceeding 13 mm. Thus, a black female athlete exhibiting LVH beyond 13 mm should be evaluated cautiously to rule out underlying pathologic conditions. Similarly, white female athletes typically do not demonstrate LVH beyond 11 mm and findings beyond this threshold should be evaluated cautiously for pathologic conditions, such as HCM.[3,6,26]

A recent addition to the literature describing athletic changes in the female heart supports that female athletes have lower LV mass (83 ± 17 g/m² vs 101 ± 21 g/m²; P<.001), as well as lower relative wall thickness (0.35 ± 0.05 vs 0.36 ± 0.05; P<.001). Additionally, though they exhibited lower absolute LV dimensions, the indexed LV measurements were greater in women (28.6 ± 2.7 mm/m² vs 27.2 ± 2.7 mm/m²; P<.001) once corrected for body surface area. Though most athletes, both men and women, had normal LV geometry, a greater proportion of women had eccentric hypertrophy compared with men (22% vs 14%; P<.001). Of additional importance, fewer women exhibited concentric hypertrophy compared with men (4% vs 15%, respectively, P<.001). None of the female athletes had a relative wall thickness greater than 0.48 or an LV mass greater than 145 g/m.² It should be noted; however, that this study only looked at white athletes.[7]

> LV wall thickness beyond 11 mm in white and 13 mm in black female athletes, should be approached cautiously and prompt further evaluation to exclude underlying pathologic conditions, such as HCM.[3,6,26]

ELECTROCARDIOGRAM DIFFERENCES

Current joint international guidelines for the interpretation of the athlete electrocardiogram (ECG) are now available, though they continue to evolve.[29] As with structural differences between male and female athletes, there are ECG differences between the 2 groups.

With regard to adolescents ages 12 to 17 years old, male athletes have been found to exhibit a greater prevalence of LVH, sinus bradycardia, and ST-segment elevation.[8]

Among 1083 healthy white athletes, there were no significant differences found between male and female athletes in regard to ECGs characterized as abnormal or normal. However, men tended to fulfill Sokolow-Lyon voltage criteria for LVH more often (42% vs 14% in women; $P<.001$). Moreover, women also rarely exhibited a QRS greater than 100 ms (3% female athletes vs 33% male athletes; $P<.001$).[7]

Compared with white athletes, black female athletes were more often found to have T-wave inversions (14% vs 2%, $P<.001$) and ST-segment elevation (11% vs 1%, $P<.001$).[6] These were particularly confined to cardiac leads V1 to V3 and were not linked to underlying HCM or arrhythmogenic RV cardiomyopathy based on further work up. This should not be mistaken for T-wave inversions seen laterally or inferiorly, which may be more likely to suggest worrisome pathologic conditions in this subgroup.

The reasoning behind ethnic differences in cardiac adaptation to exercise still remains unclear. Though vascular function and cytokine release are speculated causes for this difference, further investigation is warranted.[6]

OXYGEN CONSUMPTION PER UNIT TIME DIFFERENCES

The rate of oxygen uptake, or oxygen consumption per unit time (Vo_2), is a function of the cardiac output (heart rate times stroke volume) and arteriovenous oxygen difference. The maximum oxygen consumption (Vo_{2max}) value is used to determine the aerobic capability of the cardiovascular and respiratory systems. A link has been demonstrated between athletic performance and $Vo_{2\ max}$, particularly in endurance athletes.[30]

Maximum Vo_2 is lower in female athletes than male athletes, though differences may be less notable when adjusting for body composition.

Vo_{2max} is known to be lower in women compared with age-matched male counterparts. Multiple studies have attributed this to the differences in stroke volume between men and women, demonstrated by lower measured cardiac output in the face of similar heart rate responses during both submaximal and maximal levels of exertion.[31–33] Differences in Vo_{2max} are less drastic when results are normalized to fat-free mass, indicating that some of the gender disparity is due to body composition and increased adiposity of women. However, even when this is taken into account, female Vo_{2max} is approximately 85% of their male counterparts.[32]

CONGENITAL HEART DISEASE

Approximately 1% of the population is born with a structural congenital heart abnormality, ranging from lesions requiring surgery in the first week of life to those that are not detected until adulthood and may never cause symptoms.[34] As congenital heart surgery and catheter-based interventions have become more successful, there are more adolescents and adults with complex congenital heart disease able to participate in sports. These patients are most likely followed by a cardiologist and ideally plans for their sports participation are discussed regularly. As such, this discussion focuses on congenital heart defects that may not present until school age or later and may have implications for sports participation although they may be asymptomatic.

BICUSPID AORTIC VALVE

The presence of a bicuspid aortic valve (BAV) is the most common congenital heart defect, with an estimated prevalence between 0.5% and 2% of the population.[34,35] There is a male predominance of approximately 3 to 1.[35] BAV is often associated with left heart obstructive lesions. In fact, more than half the patients with coarctation of the aorta have been found to have BAV.[36] BAV is also commonly accompanied by dilatation of the sinuses of Valsalva, the tubular ascending aorta, or both. Although BAV or aortopathy can lead to dissection in older patients, this complication is very rare in active athletes of younger ages.[37] Of particular importance, greater than 50% of patients with Turner syndrome (a chromosomal syndrome, 45 XO, specific to women), exhibit a cardiovascular abnormality. Of these, BAV and coarctation comprise the majority.[38]

> More than 50% of patients with Turner syndrome have a cardiovascular abnormality, most common being BAV and coarctation.[38]

Physical examination findings of BAV typically include an early systolic ejection click heard best at left lower sternal border or apex. Other auscultatory findings, such as the presence of a systolic ejection murmur or diastolic murmur, will depend on the associated hemodynamic abnormalities of aortic stenosis or insufficiency.[39] Diagnosis can be made quite easily by transthoracic echocardiogram (**Fig. 2**), determining both which cusps are fused and the presence of valve dysfunction (see **Fig. 2**).

The clinical course of patients with BAV is variable and depends on the degree of valve dysfunction and/or aortic root dilation. BAV alone is typically asymptomatic, does not require activity restrictions, and can be followed every 1 to 2 years by echocardiography. However, development of aortic stenosis or insufficiency requires annual evaluation to assess need for intervention and ability to participate in athletics.[40] Development of aortic root dilation (Z-score>2 or>40 mm for adult men or >36 mm for adult women) also warrants more frequent follow-up to monitor for progression. Patients may require restriction to low-moderate levels of static and dynamic sports with avoidance of heavy weightlifting.[41] As these affected patients age, it is important that they be counseled regarding the natural history of BAV because a large percentage of these patients will require intervention as a result of progressive valve dysfunction, particularly past the fifth decade of life.[42]

HYPERTROPHIC CARDIOMYOPATHY

HCM is the most common genetic cardiovascular disease, inherited in an autosomal dominant fashion and having a prevalence of 1 in 500.[43] Most clinical studies of HCM demonstrate a male predominance of approximately 3 to 2, with some studies of

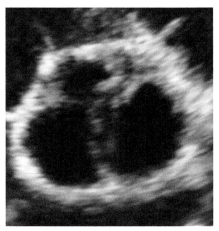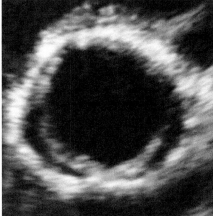

Fig. 2. Transthoracic echocardiogram (parasternal short axis view) demonstrating a BAV with right and noncoronary cusp fusion, during diastole (*left*) and during systole (*right*), demonstrating the characteristic fish-mouth appearance of an open BAV.

sudden death in athletes suggesting that HCM as a cause is 3.5 times more common among men.[22,43]

The most commonly identified cause of SCD in athletes is HCM, with a male predominance.[22] However, recent studies suggest AN-SCD may account for most SCD cases.[20,21]

HCM is characterized by a hypertrophied but nondilated left ventricle in the absence of cardiac or systemic disease that could result in LVH, such as coarctation of the aorta, aortic valve stenosis, or systemic hypertension. Hypertrophy can result in LV outflow tract (LVOT) obstruction, but obstruction may also occur at the midcavity or apex of the ventricle. The observed hypertrophy may be concentric or asymmetric, and most commonly involves the anterior septum but can be localized anywhere within the myocardium, including the apex alone.[44]

Diagnosis can be suspected due to family history, personal or family history of syncope, symptoms of heart failure, or ECG abnormalities (LVH by voltage, deep Q waves in lateral leads, inverted T waves in lateral leads) (**Fig. 3**). Physical examination is not a consistent method for diagnosis because only approximately 25% of patients with HCM will have cavity obstruction and an associated murmur. Patients with mild to moderate hypertrophy may have a normal physical examination (**Fig. 3**).[44]

Transthoracic echocardiogram is recommended for the initial evaluation of suspected HCM because this modality can visualize most segments of the ventricular myocardium. It can also identify obstruction (found in approximately 25% of patients with HCM), mitral insufficiency, and systolic anterior motion of the mitral valve.[45] CMRI has recently been identified as a useful advanced imaging technique to assist in the diagnosis in certain cases in which echocardiography proves limited because the acoustic windows are not optimal or the hypertrophy is regional and cannot be visualized. There is also added value in identifying late gadolinium enhancement (LGE), an indicator of myocardial fibrosis and scar, which may be helpful in identifying patients at increased risk of sudden death.[46]

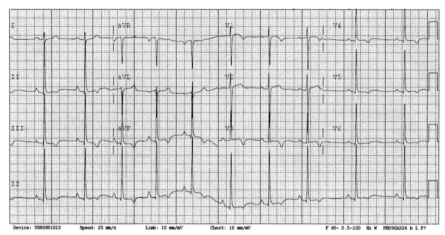

Fig. 3. A 20-year-old female distance runner with evidence of LVH by voltage and repolarization abnormalities (T-wave inversion) in the lateral leads. CMRI demonstrated concentric LVH with end-diastolic wall thickness of 13 mm, which is borderline elevated. Increased wall thickness and abnormal ECG indicate a mild form of HCM.

The clinical course of HCM can vary dramatically between patients, illustrated by age at presentation ranging from infancy to elderly. In general, there are 4 categories that can encompass complications experienced in HCM: SCD, heart failure symptoms due to obstruction, systolic or diastolic dysfunction, and atrial fibrillation.[47] Female patients have been found to progress more quickly to severe heart-failure symptoms after diagnosis but no difference has been found for risk of sudden death between male and female patients.[48] Risk of SCD is the feared complication behind the guidelines restricting high-risk individuals with HCM from participating in competitive athletics, as well as the need for placement of an implantable cardioverter defibrillator (ICD) to abort potentially lethal ventricular dysrhythmias. Several clinical features associated with increased risk of sudden death have been identified as potential indications for ICD placement[49]:

- Personal history of cardiac arrest or sustained ventricular tachycardia
- Personal history of syncope
- First-degree relative with history of SCD
- LV wall thickness greater than 30 mm
- Nonsustained ventricular tachycardia
- Abnormal blood pressure response to exercise.

Other clinical features that may modify the risk of SCD include LVOT obstruction, LGE on CMRI, and certain genetic mutations. There are not yet recommendations for ICD placement based on these factors but they may augment decision-making for a given patient.[45,46] As genetic testing has become more readily available, a population of genotype positive-phenotype negative patients has emerged. These patients are most often discovered during screening of first-degree relatives of patients with clinically evident HCM. As the name suggests, they have genetic mutations of the cardiac sarcomere that are suspected to cause disease but have no clinical or morphologic evidence of HCM. Determination of who among this group will develop a phenotype is still unclear. Other features noted on imaging, such as myocardial crypts and direct attachment of the papillary muscle to the mitral leaflet, may suggest early phenotypic development of HCM. Subsequently, most centers have advocated ongoing screening with echocardiography and ECG at routine intervals.[47,50] Case reports have also described LGE in otherwise phenotype negative patients, suggesting that CMRI may potentially become part of the screening process (**Table 1**).[51]

Though consensus guidelines do not endorse competitive sports at this time (see **Table 1**), studies are actively underway to evaluate the safety of moderate exercise in those with HCM. These include Lifestyle and Exercise in Hypertrophic Cardiomyopathy Study (LIVE-HCM; Clinicaltrials.gov identifier NCT02549664) and Randomized Exploratory Study of Exercise Training in Hypertrophic Cardiomyopathy (RESET-HCM; Clinicaltrials.gov identifier NCT01127061). It is becoming clear that many athletes with HCM at low risk may be unfairly excluded from sports participation and a shared-risk discussion with athletes and their families is evolving that may allow for future participation in select athletes.

THE MARFAN SYNDROME

Flo Hyman was arguably the best American female volleyball player until her death in 1986; she was a part the US silver medal team at the 1984 Olympic Games in Los Angeles. Hyman was playing in a match in Japan when she silently collapsed to the floor from the bench, having suddenly died from a ruptured ascending aorta. The autopsy report demonstrated evidence of a prior tear in the vessel that was healing at the time of the fatal rupture. She was unaware of her diagnosis of Marfan syndrome and subsequent need for routine cardiovascular monitoring and limitations on physical activity.[52]

The Marfan syndrome is a systemic connective tissue disorder caused by mutations in the fibrillin 1 protein, a component of the extracellular matrix. It is inherited in an autosomal dominant fashion, with an estimated incidence of 2 to 3 per 10,000.[53] Clinical reports do not describe a gender predominance regarding disease prevalence.[53,54]

The diagnostic criteria for the Marfan syndrome requires involvement of the skeletal, cardiovascular, ocular, pulmonary, or integumentary systems with or without family history or a genetic mutation of the *FBN1* gene.

Cardiovascular disease is responsible for most deaths in patients with the Marfan syndrome, although survival in recent years has been greater than in previous reports. This is likely attributed to an increase in recognition, surveillance programs, and the benefits of cardiovascular surgery.[55,56] Mitral valve prolapse (MVP) is present in approximately half of these patients with more than 25% of these displaying progression to mitral regurgitation. In 1 report, more than twice the number of female patients had progressive mitral valve dysfunction than male patients.[57] Among cardiovascular manifestations, mitral valve disease associated with Marfan syndrome uncommonly requires surgical intervention.

Table 1
Current guidelines for sports participation for patients with hypertrophic cardiomyopathy

HCM Category	2014 European Society of Cardiology Guidelines	2015 AHA/ACC Guidelines
Definite clinical HCM	No competitive sports	Class 1A sports
Definite HCM, low risk of SCD	Class 1A sports	Class 1A sports
Genotype positive- phenotype negative HCM	No sports restriction, close surveillance	No sports restriction, close surveillance

Abbreviation: AHA/ACC, American Heart Association and American College of Cardiology.

Ascending aortic dilation and dissection are the more life-threatening complications of the Marfan syndrome. They are also the most feared because, as in the case of Flo Hyman, the first symptom can be sudden death. Risk of all-cause mortality of patients with Marfan syndrome is about 4 times that of patients with a BAV but is similar to those patients with nonsyndromic thoracic aortic aneurysms.[58] Though there is no gender difference between the prevalence of aortic dilation at diagnosis or the age of onset of aortic dilation, female patients have been shown to suffer from aortic insufficiency an earlier age at diagnosis than male patients, 8.4 versus 13 years, respectively.[54]

The recommendations for athletes with the Marfan syndrome include routine noninvasive monitoring (via echocardiography, computed tomography [CT], or MRI) of aortic root dimensions every 6 to 12 months.[41] The 2015 American Heart Association and American College of Cardiology Guidelines recommend athletes participate only in class IA and IIA sports[59] (low or moderate static, or low dynamic) unless they have any complication that would then lead to more stringent limitations. These complications include

- Aortic root dilation (>40 mm or Z-score>2)
- Moderate to severe mitral regurgitation
- LV systolic dysfunction
- A family history of aortic dissection at an aortic diameter less than 50 mm.

Ultimately, the goal is to avoid isometric exercises that cause abrupt elevations in blood pressure that, in turn, result in shear stress on the vulnerable ascending aorta. These athletes should also avoid contact sports and activities in which strong blows to the chest might be sustained.[41] Aortic root replacement has been typically recommended for aortic root dimensions of 50 mm or more unless there has been rapid growth (>5 mm/y), a family history of dissection at a smaller diameter, or progressive aortic regurgitation.[60] Both beta-blockers (ie: atenolol) and angiotensin receptor blockers (ie: losartan) have been shown to be equally but modestly effective in reducing the rate of aortic dilation in patients with the Marfan syndrome.[61]

CONGENITAL CORONARY ANOMALIES

Anomalous aortic origin of a coronary artery (AAOCA) refers to either the left main coronary artery arising from the right coronary cusp or, alternatively, the right coronary artery from the left coronary cusp. Coronary artery anomalies are the second leading cause of SCD in athletes, behind HCM.[14] A recent MRI screening program in middle school students estimates an overall prevalence of AAOCA of 0.7%.[62] There is no known gender predominance although there has been a report naming congenital coronary anomalies as the leading cause of SCD in female athletes.[22]

The proposed mechanism of sudden death is thought to be from repetitive episodes of myocardial ischemia and the high-risk anatomic features. The anomalous origin of the left main coronary from right cusp portends a higher risk of SCD than anomalous origin of the right coronary artery.[63] Regardless of which variant is present, an anomalous coronary artery has intermittent reduced flow for several reasons[64,65]:

Abnormal slit-like ostium (or opening of the artery into the vessel lumen)

Acute oblique angle of the coronary that may become exaggerated during exercise due to expansion of the aorta during systole

Intramural (between the aorta and pulmonary artery) course, which may also lead to obstruction of coronary artery flow during systole as both great vessels expand (**Fig. 4**).

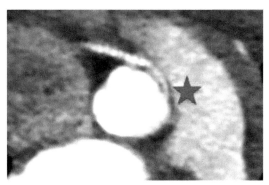

Fig. 4. A 12-year-old girl presenting with chest discomfort on exertion, CT angiogram demonstrating anomalous origin of right coronary artery from left coronary cusp (*star*) with a slit-like ostium and intramural course. She underwent an unroofing procedure and continues to have chest discomfort with activity. Exercise stress testing and myocardial perfusion scan have shown no evidence of ischemia.

AAOCA can be diagnosed by transthoracic echocardiography (see **Fig. 4**), although advanced imaging with CT or MRI angiography are often used to define the ostial anatomy and course of the vessel. Complete evaluation often includes exercise stress testing tailored to the athlete, as well as perfusion imaging, particularly if the patient is asymptomatic on presentation. These functional tests may be less helpful because they have been shown to have negative results, even in patients with AAOCA who later suffered SCD or others who presented with symptoms.[63,66] Approximately half of patients with AAOCA will report symptoms consistent with ischemia (chest pain or dyspnea with exertion, syncope, or palpitations).[17,63] Surgical management of AAOCA depends on the specific anatomy but typically involves an unroofing procedure to enlarge the coronary ostium and facilitate perfusion. Management patterns among practitioners are not consistent. Though most choose to refer for surgery when ischemia is evident (by symptoms or clinical testing), others refer based on high-risk anatomy alone. There is also no consensus regarding exercise limitations for those patients preoperatively or those who will not undergo surgery.[67,68]

Patients who do undergo the unroofing procedure will typically be restricted from exercise until they undergo an exercise stress test 3 months postoperatively.[69] There is some evidence that exercise performance does not return to baseline following the unroofing procedure and that there can be continued evidence of myocardial ischemia despite successful enlargement of the coronary ostium.[68,69] These data illustrate the ongoing controversy concerning the decision to pursue surgical correction and the postoperative testing needed to allow unlimited sports participation.

SUMMARY

SCD in athletes is a rare occurrence that has a male predilection. Recent data suggest that AN-SCD may be more common than HCM, previously identified as the most common cardiovascular cause.[21] Consensus guidelines do not endorse competitive athletics at this time; however, active studies are underway to evaluate the safety of moderate exercise in those with HCM.

HCM can usually be distinguished from athletic remodeling of the heart based on echocardiography and MRI. However, there may be cases in the gray zone that require temporary detraining and re-evaluation.

Athletic remodeling of the heart secondary to endurance sports often causes eccentric hypertrophy, that is, mild to moderate LVH with LV and RV dilatation. Conversely, strength training typically causes concentric hypertrophy and LVH without chamber dilatation.[1,23] There are several studies demonstrating differences between male and female athletic remodeling; however, the differences may be less when accounting for lean body mass.[27,28] This may also be true when comparing peak Vo_2 between genders, although in general, female athletes have 85% of the peak Vo_2 compared with their male counterparts.[32]

Other inherited cardiac conditions pertinent to athletes with exercise implications include BAV, the Marfan syndrome, and anomalous coronary arteries. The 2 latter conditions have no gender predilection.[22,54]

Future studies hold promise of further understanding of gender differences in cardiovascular remodeling and performance, as well as long-term follow-up of athletes with cardiovascular conditions.

REFERENCES

1. Morganroth J, Maron BJ, Henry WL, et al. Comparative left ventricular dimensions in trained athletes. Ann Intern Med 1975;82(4):521–4.
2. Pelliccia A, Maron BJ, Spataro A, et al. The upper limit of physiologic cardiac hypertrophy in highly trained elite athletes. N Engl J Med 1991;324(5):295–301.
3. Pelliccia A, Maron BJ, Culasso F, et al. Athlete's heart in women: echocardiographic characterization of highly trained elite female athletes. JAMA 1996;276: 211–5.
4. Pelliccia A, Cullasso F, Paolo F, et al. Physiologic left ventricular cavity dilation in elite athletes. Ann Intern Med 1999;130(1):23–31.
5. Wernstedt P, Sjöstedt C, Ekman I, et al. Adaptation of cardiac morphology and function to endurance and strength training. A comparative study using MR imaging and echocardiography in males and females. Scand J Med Sci Sports 2002;12(C):17–25.
6. Rawlins J, Carre F, Kervio G, et al. Ethnic differences in physiological cardiac adaptation to intense physical exercise in highly trained female athletes. Circulation 2010;121(9):1078–85.
7. Finocchiaro G, Dhutia H, D'Silva A, et al. Effect of sex and sporting discipline on LV adaptation to exercise. JACC Cardiovasc Imaging 2016. http://dx.doi.org/10.1016/j.jcmg.2016.08.011.
8. Pela G, Crocamo A, Li Calzi M, et al. Sex-related differences in left ventricular structure in early adolescent non-professional athletes. Eur J Prev Cardiol 2015;23(7):777–84.
9. Mitchell JH, Maron BJ, Epstein SE. 16th Bethesda conference: cardiovascular abnormalities in the athlete: recommendations regarding eligibility for competetition. J Am Coll Cardiol 1985;6(6):1186–8.
10. Maron BJ, Mitchell JH. Revised eligibility recommendations for competitive athletes with cardiovascular abnormalities. J Am Coll Cardiol 1994;24(4):848–50.
11. Pelliccia A, Zipes DP, Maron BJ. Bethesda Conference #36 and the European Society of Cardiology Consensus Recommendations revisited a comparison of U.S. and European criteria for eligibility and disqualification of competitive athletes with cardiovascular abnormalities. J Am Coll Cardiol 2008;52(24):1990–6.
12. Maron BJ, Zipes DP, Kovacs RJ. Eligibility and disqualification recommendations for competitive athletes with cardiovascular abnormalities. Circulation 2015; 132(22):e256–61.

13. Harmon KG, Asif IM, Klossner D, et al. Incidence of sudden cardiac death in national collegiate athletic association athletes. Circulation 2011;123(15):1594–600.
14. Maron BJ, Doerer JJ, Haas TS, et al. Sudden deaths in young competitive athletes analysis of 1866 deaths in the united states, 1980-2006. Circulation 2009; 119(8):1085–92.
15. Maron BJ, Haas TS, Murphy CJ, et al. Incidence and causes of sudden death in U.S. college athletes. J Am Coll Cardiol 2014;63(16):1636–43.
16. Harmon KG, Asif IM, Maleszewski JJ, et al. Incidence, cause, and comparative frequency of sudden cardiac death in national collegiate athletic association athletes a decade in review. Circulation 2015;132(1):10–9.
17. Eckart RE, Scoville SL, Campbell CL, et al. Sudden death in young adults: a 25-year review of autopsies in military recruits. Ann Intern Med 2004;141(11):829–34.
18. Bagnall RD, Weintraub RG, Ingles J, et al. A prospective study of sudden cardiac death among children and young adults. N Engl J Med 2016;374(25):2441–52.
19. Eckart RE, Shry EA, Burke AP, et al. Sudden death in young adults: an autopsy-based series of a population undergoing active surveillance. J Am Coll Cardiol 2011;58(12):1254–61.
20. Finocchiaro G, Papadakis M, Robertus JL, et al. Etiology of sudden death in sports insights from a United Kingdom regional registry. J Am Coll Cardiol 2016;67(18):2108–15.
21. Harmon KG, Drezner JA, Maleszewski JJ, et al. Pathogeneses of sudden cardiac death in national collegiate athletic association athletes. Circ Arrhythm Electrophysiol 2014;7(2):198–204.
22. Maron BJ, Haas TS, Ahluwalia A, et al. Demographics and epidemiology of sudden deaths in young competitive athletes: from the U.S. National registry. Am J Med 2016;129(11):1170–7.
23. Weiner RB, Baggish AL. Exercise-induced cardiac remodeling. Prog Cardiovasc Dis 2012;54(5):380–6.
24. Henriksen E, Landelius J, Kangro T, et al. An echocardiographic study of right and left ventricular adaptation to physical exercise in elite female orienteers. Eur Heart J 1999;20(4):309–16.
25. Sharma S, Maron BJ, Whyte G, et al. Physiologic limits of left ventricular hypertrophy in elite junior athletes: Relevance to differential diagnosis of athlete's heart and hypertrophic cardiomyopathy. J Am Coll Cardiol 2002;40(8):1431–6.
26. Whyte GP, George K, Nevill A, et al. Left ventricular morphology and function in female athletes: a meta-analysis. Int J Sports Med 2004;25(5):380–3.
27. Giraldeau G, Kobayashi Y, Finocchiaro G, et al. Gender differences in ventricular remodeling and function in college athletes, insights from lean body mass scaling and deformation imaging. Am J Cardiol 2015;116(10):1610–6.
28. Pressler A, Haller B, Scherr J, et al. Association of body composition and left ventricular dimensions in elite athletes. Eur J Prev Cardiol 2012;19(5):1194–204.
29. Sharma S, Drezner J, Baggish A, et al. International consensus standards for electrocardiographic interpretation in athletes. J Am Coll Cardiol 2017;69(8): 1058–75.
30. Foster C, Costill DL, Daniels JT, et al. Skeletal muscle enzyme activity, fiber composition, and VO2 max in relation to distance running performance. Eur J Appl Physiol 1978;39(2):73–80.
31. Wheatley CM, Snyder EM, Johnson BD, et al. Sex differences in cardiovascular function during submaximal exercise in humans. Springerplus 2014;3(1):445.
32. Ogawa T, Spina RJ, Wade HMI, et al. Effects of aging, sex, and physical training cardiovascular responses to exercise. Circulation 1992;86(2):494–504.

33. Higginbotham MB, Morris KG, Coleman RE, et al. Sex-related differences in the normal cardiac response to upright exercise. Circulation 1984;70(3):357–66.

34. Hoffman JIE, Kaplan S. The incidence of congenital heart disease. J Am Coll Cardiol 2002;39(12):1890–900.

35. Basso C, Boschello M, Perrone C, et al. An echocardiographic survey of primary school children for bicuspid aortic valve. Am J Cardiol 2004;93(5):661–3.

36. Roos-Hesselink JW, Schölzel BE, Heijdra RJ, et al. Aortic valve and aortic arch pathology after coarctation repair. Heart 2003;89:1074–7.

37. Larson EW, Edwards WD. Risk factors for aortic dissection: a necropsy study of 161 cases. Am J Cardiol 1984;53(6):849–55.

38. Sybert VP. Cardiovascular malformations and complications in Turner syndrome. Pediatrics 1998;101(1):E11.

39. Siu SC, Silversides CK. Bicuspid aortic valve disease. J Am Coll Cardiol 2010; 55(25):2789–800.

40. Bonow RO, Nishimura RA, Thompson PD, et al. Eligibility and disqualification recommendations for competitive athletes with cardiovascular abnormalities: task force 5: valvular heart disease: a scientific statement from the American Heart Association and American College of Cardiology. Circulation 2015;132(22):e292–7.

41. Braverman AC, Harris KM, Kovacs RJ, et al. Eligibility and disqualification recommendations for competitive athletes with cardiovascular abnormalities: task force 7: aortic diseases, including Marfan syndrome: a scientific statement from the American Heart Association and American College of Cardiology. J Am Coll Cardiol 2015;66(21):2398–405.

42. Michelena HI, Desjardins VA, Avierinos JF, et al. Natural history of asymptomatic patients with normally functioning or minimally dysfunctional bicuspid aortic valve in the community. Circulation 2008;117(21):2776–84.

43. Semsarian C, Ingles J, Maron MS, et al. New perspectives on the prevalence of hypertrophic cardiomyopathy. J Am Coll Cardiol 2015;65(12):1249–54.

44. Maron BJ, Maron MS. Hypertrophic cardiomyopathy. J Am Med Assoc 2002; 287(10):1308–20.

45. Elliott PM, Gimeno JR, Tomé MT, et al. Left ventricular outflow tract obstruction and sudden death risk in patients with hypertrophic cardiomyopathy. Eur Heart J 2006;27(16):1933–41.

46. Green JJ, Berger JS, Kramer CM, et al. Prognostic value of late gadolinium enhancement in clinical outcomes for hypertrophic cardiomyopathy. JACC Cardiovasc Imaging 2012;5(4):370–7.

47. Gersh BJ, Maron BJ, Bonow RO, et al. 2011 ACCF/AHA guideline for the diagnosis and treatment of hypertrophic cardiomyopathy. J Thorac Cardiovasc Surg 2011;142(6):e153–203.

48. Olivotto I, Maron MS, Adabag AS, et al. Gender-related differences in the clinical presentation and outcome of hypertrophic cardiomyopathy. J Am Coll Cardiol 2005;46(3):480–7.

49. Tracy CM, Epstein AE, Darbar D, et al. 2012 ACCF/AHA/HRS focused update of the 2008 guidelines for device-based therapy of cardiac rhythm abnormalities: a report of the American College of Cardiology Foundation/American Heart Association task force on practice guidelines. J Am Coll Cardiol 2012;60(14):1297–313.

50. Maron BJ, Yeates L, Semsarian C. Clinical challenges of genotype positive (+)-phenotype negative (-) family members in hypertrophic cardiomyopathy. Am J Cardiol 2011;107(4):604–8.

51. Rowin EJ, Maron MS, Lesser JR, et al. CMR with late gadolinium enhancement in genotype positive-phenotype negative hypertrophic cardiomyopathy. JACC Cardiovasc Imaging 2012;5(1):119–22.
52. Demak R. Marfan syndrome: a silent killer. Sport Illus 1986;30–5.
53. Judge DP, Dietz HC. Marfan's syndrome. Lancet 2005;366(9501):1965–76.
54. Mueller GC, Stark V, Steiner K, et al. Impact of age and gender on cardiac pathology in children and adolescents with Marfan syndrome. Pediatr Cardiol 2013; 34(4):991–8.
55. Nichol KP, Cherry JD. Life expectancy and causes of death in the Marfan syndrome. N Engl J Med 1967;277(13):667–72.
56. Silverman DI, Burton KJ, Gray J, et al. Life expectancy in the Marfan syndrome. Am J Cardiol 1994;75:157–60.
57. Pyeritz RE, Wappel MA. Mitral valve dysfunction in the Marfan syndrome. Clinical and echocardiographic study of prevalence and natural history. Am J Med 1983; 74(5):797–807.
58. Sherrah AG, Andvik S, Van Der Linde D, et al. Nonsyndromic thoracic aortic aneurysm and dissection outcomes with Marfan syndrome versus bicuspid aortic valve aneurysm. J Am Coll Cardiol 2016;67(6):618–26.
59. Braverman AC, Harris KM, Kovacs RJ, et al. Eligibility and disqualification recommendations for competitive athletes with cardiovascular abnormalities: task force 7: aortic diseases, including Marfan syndrome: a scientific statement from the American Heart Association and American College of Cardiology. Circulation 2015;132(22):e303–9.
60. Milewicz DM. Treatment of aortic disease in patients with Marfan syndrome. Circulation 2005;111(11):e150–7.
61. Lacro RV, Dietz HC, Sleeper LA, et al. Atenolol versus losartan in children and young adults with Marfan's syndrome. N Engl J Med 2014;371(22):2061–71.
62. Angelini P. Novel imaging of coronary artery anomalies to assess their prevalence, the causes of clinical symptoms, and the risk of sudden cardiac death. Circ Cardiovasc Imaging 2014;7(4):747–54.
63. Basso C, Maron BJ, Corrado D, et al. Clinical profile of congenital coronary artery anomalies with origin from the wrong aortic sinus leading to sudden death in young competitive athletes. J Am Coll Cardiol 2000;35(6):1493–501.
64. Basso C, Frescura C, Corrado D, et al. Congenital heart disease and sudden death in the young. Hum Pathol 1995;26(10):1065–72. Available at: http://www.ncbi.nlm.nih.gov/pubmed/7557938.
65. Frescura C, Basso C, Thiene G, et al. Anomalous origin of coronary arteries and risk of sudden death: A study based on an autopsy population of congenital heart disease. Hum Pathol 1998;29(7):689–95.
66. Brothers JA, McBride MG, Seliem MA, et al. Evaluation of myocardial ischemia after surgical repair of anomalous aortic origin of a coronary artery in a series of pediatric patients. J Am Coll Cardiol 2007;50(21):2078–82.
67. Brothers J, Gaynor JW, Paridon S, et al. Anomalous aortic origin of a coronary artery with an interarterial course: understanding current management strategies in children and young adults. Pediatr Cardiol 2009;30(7):911–21.
68. Brothers JA, McBride MG, Marino BS, et al. Exercise performance and quality of life following surgical repair of anomalous aortic origin of a coronary artery in the pediatric population. J Thorac Cardiovasc Surg 2009;137(2):380–4.
69. Molossi S, Grenier M. The management of athletes with congenital heart disease. Clin Sports Med 2015;34(3):551–70.

Nutritional Aspects of the Female Athlete

Kelly A. Rossi, MS, RD, CSSD

KEYWORDS

- Energy • Macronutrients • Iron • Calcium • Vitamin D • Hydration
- Gastrointestinal (GI) • Supplements

KEY POINTS

- Female athletes report a lower energy availability (EA) than male athletes. Low EA, in turn, may affect menstrual cycle, injury risk, and performance.
- Female athletes may require individualized strategies for carbohydrate and protein timing with dosage based on hormonal fluctuations. However, current research advocates individualizing recommendations based on body weight, training intensity, and duration.
- Female athletes exhibit low levels of many of the essential micronutrients, suggesting that recommendation levels may be too low for active women.
- Although research implies that hormonal variations in women do not alter fluid or electrolyte needs enough to alter current recommendations, further research is needed.
- Other nutritional concerns, such as runner's gut, celiac disease, eating disorders, supplements, and the microbiome, all present intriguing areas of interest for additional research in female athletes.

NUTRITIONAL CONCERNS

Every athlete has specific needs based on his or her individual sex, size, sport, exercise intensity, duration of activity, phase of training, and even the season in which the sport is played. Nutritionally, the female athlete is unique in many ways, with needs that may vary based on hormonal fluctuations related to the menstrual cycle. This article provides an overview of the distinct nutritional needs and concerns of the physically active female, including energy availability (EA), macronutrient needs, micronutrient needs, hydration, supplements, and other nutritional issues, such as gastrointestinal (GI) issues, eating disorders, the microbiome, and celiac disease (CD). Although there is some research focusing specifically on the female athlete

Disclosure Statement: The author has nothing to disclose.
Department of Athletics, University of Virginia, 290 Massie Road, PO Box 400845, Charlottesville, VA 22904, USA
E-mail address: kar7k@virginia.edu

Clin Sports Med 36 (2017) 627–653
http://dx.doi.org/10.1016/j.csm.2017.05.007
0278-5919/17/© 2017 Elsevier Inc. All rights reserved.

and her exceptional nutritional concerns, further gender-specific exploration is needed in all areas.

Energy Needs

Energy intake plays an important role for the female athlete. Although female athletes require less overall energy than male athletes, research shows that many come up short of their energy needs, putting them at higher risk for injury, menstrual dysfunction, and decreased performance. EA is the amount of energy available for the metabolic processes of the body after energy is used for exercise, and normalized for fat-free mass (FFM):

EA = Energy intake (EI) – Energy expenditure (EE) per kilogram of FFM[1]

The threshold for low EA has been defined as 30 kcal/kg FFM/d, but more research is needed to validate this number and its long-term implications.[2] The multiple causes of low EA include disordered eating, intentional but rational efforts to decrease body weight (BW) for sport, and the unintentional failure to meet energy requirements. Some issues, such as time management, food availability, and lack of nutritional knowledge, also may affect EA.[1] On the other hand, factors may increase energy *needs* above expected levels, making it more difficult for female athletes to meet their requirements: cold, fear, stress, heat, altitude, injuries, medications, and hormonal changes.[3]

Inadequate EI and nutrition may lead to decreased performance in addition to affecting growth and physiologic development in female athletes. A recent survey found that 45% of recreational female athletes were classified as "at risk" for low EA, with those in individual sports at a higher risk for low EA than those in team sports.[4] Koutedakis and Jamurtas[5] reported that female dancers consume less than 70% of recommended daily energy needs. A study of female soccer players also supports the theory that female athletes underfuel their bodies, with consumption of 500 fewer kilocalories than their estimated needs.[6] Almost twice as many adolescent female swimmers had insufficient EI compared with controls in a 3-year study assessing bone health.[7] The swimmers displayed negative bone density z-scores, likely attributed to inadequate energy and/or calcium intake. Conversely, Coutinho and colleagues[8] found that female athletes had a higher EI than the general recommendations by the Academy of Nutrition and Dietetics; however, these provided recommendations may have been inaccurate relative to the needs of athletes.

The effect of ovarian suppression on female athletes with low EA has been studied. Female swimmers exhibiting low EA with secondary ovarian suppression had impaired performance (decreased by 9.8%), whereas the females with cyclic menstrual function showed an 8.2% improvement in performance.[9] Total triiodothyronine (TT3) was 19% lower in ovarian-suppressed females and EA was 90% lower than their eumenorrheic counterparts. Performance also worsened if the energy deficit was not corrected. This was the first study of its kind.

Energy density (ED), defined as "…energy (kcal) per gram weight of food," affects EA.[10] A low-ED diet consists of a high volume of food with low energy content.[10] Consumption of a low-ED diet (ie, fruits, vegetables, high-fiber grains) enhances weight management and satiety, yet has been associated with problems such as exercise-associated menstrual dysfunction (ExMD) and low EA relative to EI.[10] Recent research shows that 44% of female athletes with ExMD who consumed a low-ED diet failed to meet the energy demands of their sport.[10] Reed and colleagues[11] also reported that active females with ExMD exhibited lower ED diets than those with regular menstrual cycles. In addition, subjects also had lower resting EE, EI, and consumed more vegetables, fat-free condiments, and noncaloric beverages than their counterparts. The greater consumption of low energy-dense foods may be allowing these women to consume fewer calories due to increased satiety. Additional research is necessary to further clarify the effects of low-ED diets on the menstrual function and EA of female athletes.

Overall, female athletes report a lower EA than male athletes; at a higher risk are those who restrict EI. Energy restriction may be due to disordered eating, high energy demands of the sport, or a low-ED diet. Regardless, low EA may affect menstrual cycle, injury risk, and performance, and continued research is needed to support the current data.

Macronutrients

Carbohydrates

Carbohydrates are a food often feared by many female athletes; however, they are essential in hormonal balance, providing energy for both aerobic and anaerobic metabolism, as well as fuel for the brain and central nervous system. Carbohydrate needs for athletes vary based on changing activity levels, as well as training intensity, duration, and frequency.[12] Heavy training day needs are met by adding carbohydrate-based meals and snacks around workouts to encourage better performance and recovery.[12]

Burke and colleagues[12] coined the term *carbohydrate availability* to describe the carbohydrate content of an athlete's diet. It is used in defining how well an athlete's carbohydrate intake meets the fuel cost of training, versus the previous terms *low-carbohydrate diet* or *high-carbohydrate diet*. *Carbohydrate availability* is expressed relative to the athlete's training, not the absolute grams of carbohydrate ingested. For example, one would have low carbohydrate availability if she were not meeting the fuel needs of her training on a specific day, even if her total intake of carbohydrate in grams may seem high. This new definition supports the changes in carbohydrate guidelines recommended by Burke and colleagues[13] in 2004, suggesting that needs be based on the athlete's body mass (g/kg BW) versus the percentage of total EI. Carbohydrate targets should be individualized to the athlete's training and dietary goals, and how such changes alter their training experience. Most evidence suggests that it may be beneficial for female athletes to focus on maintaining high carbohydrate availability in their diet during training, resulting in power gains, increased time to fatigue, and less physiologic fatigue.[14] Other research found no differences in time to exhaustion or rate of perceived exertion with carbohydrate intake, specifically during the mid-follicular phase of the menstrual cycle.[14] However, subjects were consuming only 6.5 g/kg per day carbohydrate versus the recommended 8 g/kg per day.[14] More research is needed to assess possible differences in the needs of female compared with male athletes, although individualizing recommendations for each athlete will allow somewhat more gender-specific recommendations.[15] Current daily carbohydrate needs based on training are separated into 4 categories (**Table 1**).

Multiple studies support the notion that female athletes fail to meet their carbohydrate needs. The study by Gibson and colleagues[6] showed that 51.5% of female soccer players consumed <5 g/kg per day carbohydrate. Burke and colleagues[15] reported that female athletes consume 30% less carbohydrate per kilogram of BW than their male counterparts in the same sport, and also underfuel compared with carbohydrate recommendations. Tarnopolsky and colleagues[16] also indicated that female athletes had lower energy and carbohydrate intakes than male athletes relative to body mass, and required an increase in EI by a third to enhance glycogen storage. Additionally, Masson and Lamarche[17] reported that both male and female

Table 1
Daily carbohydrate needs

	Training Level	g/kg BW/d
Light	Low-intensity or skill-based activity	3–5
Moderate	1 h/d	5–7
High	Endurance: 1–3 h/d of moderate to high-intensity activity	6–10
Very high	Exercise lasting >4 h/d; moderate to high-intensity	8–12

Data from Burke L, Hawley J, Wong S, et al. Carbohydrates for training and competition. J Sports Sci 2011;29:S17–27.

nonelite multisport athletes failed to meet carbohydrate recommendations, with only 45.7% of athletes consuming optimal carbohydrate intakes.

For females, especially during the low estrogen phase of the menstrual cycle, carbohydrates are particularly important to support the increase in glycogen utilization. Higher glycogen storage and lower carbohydrate oxidation is seen during the luteal phase (increased circulating estrogen and progesterone) of the menstrual cycle compared with the follicular phase (suppressed progesterone and late surge of estrogen).[14] Therefore, increased attention on carbohydrate loading during the follicular phase is important for increasing glycogen storage.[18] Some research reports that higher estrogen in females spares hepatic glycogen stores by decreasing total glucose oxidation during exercise, making carbohydrate loading less essential during the luteal phase.[14] The ability of the female body to preserve muscle glycogen and favor lipid oxidation supports the notion that females may perform better in longer distance events (>66 km).[19]

To reiterate, carbohydrate replacement during exercise should be specific to the training intensity and duration. Previous recommendations were based on research indicating that carbohydrate oxidation happens at a rate of 1 g/min.[20] Current carbohydrate recommendations for training can be found in **Table 2**.

Research supports improved performance with higher intakes of carbohydrate, especially multiple transportable carbohydrates (MTCs). MTCs are a combination of saccharides that use different glucose transporters, reducing intestinal carbohydrate and GI symptoms.[21] Consuming MTCs instead of glucose alone allows for higher rates of carbohydrate oxidation.[14] Mouth rinsing with carbohydrates is another strategy used specifically for shorter-duration activity. This triggers the central nervous system to sense the presence of carbohydrate in the mouth, and may enhance performance by 2% to 3% through improved pacing and an increased sense of well-being.[14] Carbohydrate oxidation also may be maximized with nighttime consumption of chocolate milk for early morning activity, a finding found in female athletes.[22] Although there were

Table 2
Carbohydrate needs during training

<45 min	Nothing additional
45–75 min	Small amounts CHO; mouth rinse
1.0–2.5 h	30–60 g/h
>2.5–3.0 h	Up to 90 g/h

Data from Burke L, Dziedzic C. Carbohydrate requirements for the female athlete. In: Beals K, editor. Nutrition and the female athlete. Boca Raton, London, New York: CRC Press; 2013. p. 29.

no significant performance effects, next-morning resting and exercise metabolism favored carbohydrate oxidation. All of these strategies need additional female-specific research.

During the recovery phase of training, female athletes appear to replenish glycogen stores much the same as male athletes when carbohydrate intake is matched to body mass.[23] For general refueling of carbohydrates, the recommendation is to consume 1.0 to 1.2 g/kg per hour for the first 4 hours when an athlete has 2 fuel-demanding sessions within 8 hours of each other.[12] When recovery time is >24 hours, the athlete can choose the timing and types of carbohydrate based on her preferences and what is functional.[14] In this situation, research shows no difference in glycogen resynthesis with solids versus liquids or with large meals versus smaller, more frequent meals.[14] Although the foremost benefit of consuming protein after exercise is to promote muscle protein synthesis, protein also may promote higher glycogen storage in the early stages of recovery if carbohydrate intake is low (<1 g/kg).[14,24]

Glycogen supercompensation When planning fueling for competition, carbohydrate loading (glycogen supercompensation) could prove beneficial in events lasting longer than 90 minutes. Although Tarnopolsky and colleagues reported that females were not responsive to carbohydrate loading, a follow-up study in 2001 noted that women exhibit no difference in the ability to glycogen load compared with men when provided with carbohydrate and energy amounts relative to lean body mass.[14,16] General guidelines suggest that carbohydrate loading is optimal for female athletes at a rate of 10 to 12 g/kg BW/d for the 36 to 48 hours leading up to an event.[12] For events less than 90 minutes, 7 to 12 g/kg BW for the 24 hours leading up to the event is ideal, with a preference for low fiber/low residue carbohydrates. The recommendation is to consume 1 to 4 g/kg BW of carbohydrate for the 1 to 4 hours directly preceding an athletic event.[12]

Training low The idea of *training low* (consuming a low-carbohydrate diet to enhance training-induced adaptations) has become popular in the world of athletics. However, the risks and benefits are important to understand. The concept began with studies indicating that exercising in a glycogen-depleted state enhances fat metabolism.[14] The goal is to choose specific training sessions to *train low* but increase carbohydrate for competition, and *compete high*.[25] The aim of training low is to increase lipid oxidation rates and mitochondrial enzyme activity, enhance exercise capacity, and spare glycogen.[25] There are multiple ways to implement the train low strategy:

1. Training after an overnight fast of more than 6 hours
2. Withholding carbohydrates between 2 training sessions
3. Avoiding carbohydrates in the few hours of recovery
4. Sleeping low/training low (undertaking a carbohydrate-depleting training session at night with an overnight fast, followed by a training session in the morning)[14,26]

However, training low is not without its risks. It can cause reduced training intensities and inability to oxidize endogenous carbohydrate. It also fails to provide a consistently synergistic increase in performance in conjunction with the enhanced lipid oxidation and metabolic enzyme activity.[14,27] Muscle protein breakdown (MPB) also increases with low glycogen availability during exercise.[28] Therefore, the athlete should aim to include optimal protein intake surrounding training if she plans to attempt this approach.[29] To offset the intensity issue, a CHO mouth rinse and/or the intake of caffeine before exercise has proven beneficial.[30] Another risk of training low is infection and illness, as carbohydrates prevent the immunosuppression caused by intense exercise.[31] Implementing the *train low* strategy in training sessions that are familiar to the athlete, and not during supramaximal, prolonged workouts will minimize the risks.[25] The athlete must take care in deciding where and when to implement the strategy, and understand that training low does not mean chronic low-carbohydrate intake, but selectively decreasing carbohydrate intake around times of consistent, high carbohydrate intake.[26] Future research will help elucidate the specifics of which type of *train low* method provides the best possible outcomes, where in the training cycle it should be implemented, and how males and females might respond differently. Another low-carbohydrate strategy is the fat-adapted/ketogenic diet, which is discussed in the fat/lipids section.

Fat/lipids
Dietary fat is known for its role in reducing inflammation, cellular membrane formation, absorption of fat-soluble vitamins, maintaining hormonal balance, and energy metabolism.[3] In female athletes, lipid utilization surrounding exercise differs from male athletes. Research shows that women have a lower respiratory exchange ratio (RER) than men, using more fat during exercise. Females demonstrate greater lipolytic activity during prolonged, moderate exercise than males with similar fat mass and training levels.[32] Estrogen enhances lipid oxidation during exercise, which provides an increase in free fatty acids to the exercising female athlete.[32] When males were supplemented with 17-β-estradiol they also exhibited a lower RER, supporting the role of estrogen in fat metabolism.[33] Sarafian and colleagues[34] also supported the gender difference in substrate oxidation during low-intensity, isometric exercise, reporting that female subjects demonstrated increased fat oxidation, whereas males increased both fat and carbohydrate oxidation. Fat oxidation is higher in females even with high glycogen availability.[3]

One theory on increased fat oxidation in females during exercise is their higher intramuscular triglycerides (IMTG) stores. Most research supports gender-based differences in the use of IMTGs during prolonged, moderate-intensity exercise.[32] Although some research has shown that males use intramyocellular lipids to a greater extent than females during endurance exercise, there is a possibility that the male subjects began these studies in a more trained state than their female counterparts.[33,35] Dietary fat intake may also have an influence on fat oxidation,[31,32,36] although most gender comparison studies demonstrate no significant difference based on macronutrient composition of the diet.[31] Vogt and colleagues[36] reported that although duathletes' IMTG stores doubled and lipids contributed a significantly greater percentage of total energy demands on a 5-week high-fat diet, endurance performance remained the same. Research also suggests that there are notable gender differences in fat oxidation due to a higher percentage of type I muscle fibers in females, who exhibit a greater expression of fatty acid transport proteins.[33] In support of this theory, women have shown higher fatty acid transport protein levels.[32] With higher fat stores and the ability to oxidize fat more efficiently during endurance events, women may be better suited for endurance events than their male counterparts. More research is needed focusing expressly on the possible advantage female athletes have in endurance competition.

Conversely, the *postexercise* mobilization of fatty acids is lower in females compared with males, which may contribute to why women have a higher fat mass than males.[32] One study showed that postexercise lipolysis rates in women remained elevated for 3 hours, whereas men presented with elevated lipid oxidation into the second day postexercise.[32] Other research also supported females' enhanced ability for gluco-regulation after exercise compared with males, reducing the need for lipolysis in females.[32]

Fat-adapted/low-carbohydrate high-fat/ketogenic diet Another fueling strategy is the fat-adapted/low-carbohydrate high-fat (LCHF)/ketogenic diet. These terms will be used interchangeably, although there may be slight variations in their definition based on the literature referenced. Because fat is an abundant and more available energy source in endurance-trained athletes, some researchers theorized the use of chronic fat adaptation with a very high-fat, moderate protein, low-carbohydrate diet.[37] Similar benefits and concerns are present with the LCHF diet as with the *training low* strategy discussed previously. LCHF diets may be useful in ultra-endurance events when energy stores may be limited, increasing rates of fat oxidation. Recent research demonstrated that rates of muscle glycogen utilization and repletion were similar in LCHF diets compared with a high-carbohydrate diet.[37] However, the impact of an LCHF diet on performance was not assessed, which is the most critical outcome for athletes.[37] Another recent study reported a negative impact on performance (endurance capacity, peak power, and faster exhaustion) with a ketogenic diet, although this research was done in healthy adults, not athletes.[38] Arguably, there are more disadvantages than advantages with athletes using ketogenic diets, including reduced metabolic flexibility, decreased training intensities, immunosuppression, loss of lean mass, lack of performance improvement, and the inability to use carbohydrates as an efficient fuel source during exercise.[3] If an endurance athlete requires the ability to sprint at the end of a race, following a high-fat approach may prevent her from tapping into her carbohydrate stores quickly enough.

However, limiting fat excessively can have negative effects on athletes as well, including reduced EA, increased inflammation, and depletion of fat-soluble vitamins. Because females have a greater ability to store and use fat during exercise, they may benefit from a higher fat intake after exercise to replenish IMTG stores (possibly 30%–40% of energy).[33] Some research shows that fat intake was below recommended levels in female athletes.[6] In general, athletes should keep their fat intake above 20% of EI to ensure adequate intake of fat-soluble vitamins and essential fatty acids.[3]

In summary, differences in fat oxidation between males and females may be present due to hormonal fluctuations, IMTG stores, or differences in type I muscle fibers. However, more research is needed to assess the effect of these differences on performance and how female athletes may benefit, specifically in endurance events. Although there are some benefits of using a fat-adapted diet, research assessing the effect on performance outcomes is still lacking. Currently, the risks seem to outweigh the benefits.

Protein

Protein is a macronutrient essential for protein synthesis, as well as immune function and tissue growth, maintenance, and repair.[39] When looking at general guidelines for protein intake, research does not differentiate between male and female athletes. Some studies suggested that protein needs are met by following the recommended dietary allowance (RDA), but the use of nitrogen balance in this research may underestimate optimal protein intake for athletes.[40] Other research has shown that male endurance athletes need more protein than the RDA, thus, female athletes may also benefit from higher protein intakes than their nonactive counterparts.[41–43] Higher protein intakes are also important to preserve lean mass if an athlete exhibits low EA, is recovering from injury, or for short periods during intense training.[44] A level of 2.0 g/kg BW/d in these situations has been shown to prevent loss of FFM.[45] Daily recommended ranges for protein are 1.2 to 2.0 g/kg BW/d. Scientists no longer categorize athletes based on strength versus endurance, as needs should be individualized and periodized based on training.[3] Carbohydrate and EA are also important factors in assessing the protein requirements of an athlete, as matching carbohydrate and EI to EE will ensure that protein is not oxidized for fuel, preserving it for lean mass growth and repair.[46]

Female athletes generally consume optimal quantities of protein, unlike the typical deficits found in energy, fat, and carbohydrate intake.[47,48] However, female athletes in "thin build" sports are often at risk for low protein intake due to the presence of low EA.[32,48] Additionally, Hinton and colleagues[48] found that most female subjects consumed less than the recommended amounts for both carbohydrate and protein relative to BW. Protein intake in female soccer players in one study was below recommended levels, with 27.3% of subjects consuming less than 1.2 g/kg protein.[6] Conversely, protein intake and distribution patterns were examined in a recent study in male and female athletes across strength, endurance, and team sports, and it was found that females consumed greater than 1.2 g/kg of protein daily.[49] The conflicting evidence implies that additional research is needed to define the true prevalence of inadequate protein intake in female athletes.

It has been found that females use less protein than males both at rest and during exercise, likely regulated by hepatic activation differences in branched-chain 2-oxoacid dehydrogenase.[32] Protein catabolism during exercise in females is higher in the luteal phase compared with the follicular phase, which may be partially due to higher circulating progesterone or a reduced estrogen/progesterone ratio.[50] Administration of gonadotropin-releasing hormone agonist to induce ovarian suppression also supported the influence of estrogen/ovarian hormones on increased protein breakdown and synthesis.[51] However, these effects seem to be insignificant when carbohydrate was supplemented during exercise.[52] Thus, a hormonal influence on metabolism may be secondary to substrate availability and exercise, although additional research is critical for understanding these effects.

During recovery, muscle protein synthesis (MPS) is similar in men and women, although females have higher MPB rates, thus a greater likelihood of negative net protein balance than males.[39] However, some research indicates that MPS and MPB are similar at rest and after exercise in *young* males and females.[53] Throughout postexercise recovery, MPS and strength are optimized when consuming 10 g essential amino acids within the 2 hours after exercise.[3] This amounts to approximately 15 to 25 g of high biological value protein for most athletes, or 0.25 to 0.3 g/kg BW.[54] Josse and colleagues[55] detailed that females consuming milk (protein and carbohydrates) versus carbohydrate alone, immediately and 1 hour after exercise, had greater gains in lean mass, strength, serum 25-hydroxyvitamin D, and increased fat loss. The benefit of protein consumption after exercise continues for the 24-hour period after activity, showing dose rather than time as most imperative in maximizing MPS postexercise.[56] Intermediate dosing with 20 g protein every 3 hours increased MPS after exercise more than 8 doses of 10 g, or 2 doses of 40 g.[56] In addition to focusing on timing and dosage of protein after exercise, Phillips[57] also discussed the benefit of choosing quickly digested proteins high in leucine and the essential amino acids to optimize MPS. Arnal and colleagues[58] reported that the patterns of protein consumption have no effect on protein retention in young women, although a pulse pattern of protein feeding (feeding protein in multiple meals) increased protein retention in elderly women. Protein dose per meal relative to BW shows some benefit in individualizing protein needs by gender and athlete. A per-meal dose of 0.25 g/kg BW protein is what current literature states will optimally stimulate MPS.[59] Recent evidence also supports that consumption of protein at night (complemented with resistance exercise) enhances muscle mass and strength gains.[60] Whey protein is still the most superior choice, although most of the protein research was completed in men.[57]

A continued push for research examining the effect of protein type, dosing, and timing on female athletes is necessary. Although current scientific evidence suggests that the differences are too small to alter protein recommendations specifically for women, further investigation into the female athlete's response to changes in sex hormones surrounding exercise, and how nutritional modifications might affect protein levels and performance are essential.

Micronutrients

Micronutrients are a crucial part of an athlete's diet. The stress of exercise may increase the need for some micronutrients if EI is suboptimal or certain foods are restricted.[3] Gibson and colleagues[6] reported that female soccer players consumed suboptimal intakes of iron, calcium, folate, vitamin E, pantothenic acid, and vitamin D, showing depleted serum levels. This section will explore micronutrients and their effect on female athletes. As you will see throughout this section, there is a paucity of data investigating the effects of individual micronutrient levels and dosing effects on female athletes. More research is needed in all areas.

Iron

Optimal iron stores are important to support high aerobic capacity in the female athlete.[61] Low iron has been shown to negatively impact performance due to the impairment of muscle function, oxidative metabolism, and work capacity.[62] Other consequences of low iron important to the female athlete are lowered nonspecific immunity, impaired cognition, and reduced high-density lipoproteins (HDLs).[61] Although the RDA is the same for both female athletes and nonathletes (**Table 3**), iron losses in athletes are increased by 30% to 70% due to physical activity, suggesting a need for higher iron requirements in female athletes.[61] Rowers with lower iron status exhibited decreased performance times and reduced ability to practice at optimal levels, ultimately affecting racing performance.[63] They also reported lower Vo_{2max} scores and lower energetic efficiency.[63]

Athletes in general are at an increased risk of iron deficiency anemia (IDA) or iron deficiency without anemia (IDNA) due to the high stress workload of sport, iron loss through sweat and urine, visceral ischemia, GI losses from nonsteroidal anti-inflammatory drugs (NSAIDs) overuse, and foot-strike hemolysis in endurance training.[61,62] Also common in athletes of both sexes is "athlete's pseudo-anemia," or the acute expansion in plasma volume due to heavy training.[64] This presents with low hemoglobin (Hb) levels accompanied by normal serum ferritin on laboratory workup. Female athletes in particular have other considerations that may compound their risk of low iron levels, including low dietary iron intake, vegan/vegetarian diets, or heavy menstrual bleeding.[61] Looking at the athlete as a whole and considering risk factors helps determine risk of IDA/IDNA.

Table 3	
Recommended dietary allowance for iron: females	
Years of Age	**mg/d**
19–50	18
≥51	8
Pregnant	27
Lactating	9

Data from Hinton P. Trace minerals of concern for female athletes: iron and zinc. In: Beals K, editor. Nutrition and the female athlete; 2013. p. 96.

To complicate matters more, there is a lack of consensus on definitions surrounding iron assessment laboratory measurements, particularly that of ferritin. Currently cut-offs range from less than 10 to less than 35 ng/mL to indicate low levels.[3] Some researchers use levels of $\leq$25 ng/mL to define IDNA, and define IDA as Hb levels less than 12 g/dL in conjunction with ferritin levels less than 12 to 20 ng/mL.[62–64] Optimal blood values to define IDNA and IDA still remain to be clarified.

Recent data suggest a prevalence of 56% to 60% of female athletes presenting with IDNA and 20% with IDA.[62] These percentages are higher than previous research, attributable to an increased training volume and multiple daily workouts affecting iron absorption, as well as the other risk factors discussed previously. However, disagreement on prevalence numbers still remains among scientists.

Research also shows that low EI and low intake of high iron-containing foods, such as heme foods (ie, beef, chicken, pork), may affect iron status.[61] Thus, the high prevalence of IDNA and IDA in female athletes may be partially attributed to low dietary iron intake. Baranauskas and colleagues[65] found that female endurance athletes consumed low iron (36% lower than recommended levels), and multiple studies have shown that female swimmers also displayed low iron intakes (65%–82% of subjects).[7]

Another important contributor to iron balance/status is the presence of a peptide hormone called hepcidin. As training levels increase, inflammation escalates and enhances hepcidin production, causing impaired iron uptake.[61] Peak hepcidin levels are seen 3 to 6 hours after exercise. The timing of iron supplementation may affect hepcidin levels, with higher iron doses causing hepcidin to increase acutely and reduce endogenous iron uptake.[66] Because hepcidin levels remain high for up to 24 hours after supplementation (with doses >60 mg), alternating days of iron supplementation are recommended to enhance absorption.[66] This approach may also decrease GI issues. Optimal absorption of iron in nonanemic young females occurs with a dosage between 40 and 80 mg/d.[66] Additionally, even partial repletion of iron stores will have a positive effect, although longer-term studies are needed on hepcidin.

Although the International Olympic Committee recommends periodic assessment of iron status in athletes, only 43% of National Collegiate Athletic Association (NCAA) Division I institutions complete these screenings.[61] Individual circumstances also may skew the accuracy of blood draws, including injury, illness, and time of last training bout. Furthermore, as previously noted, endurance training also can cause "pseudo-sports anemia" or dilutional anemia.[61] It is important to be aware of all possible issues that may affect the accuracy of iron assessment.

Vitamin D

Vitamin D has gained a lot of attention over the past decade for its role in bone strength, immune health, and its likely role in the maintenance of athletic performance. There is conflicting research and much debate among scientists over the ideal RDA and the optimal dosage of supplementation, and whether or not supplementation is needed at all. Vitamin D is a prohormone that supports many other systems in the body. With limited amounts of vitamin D occurring naturally in food, most is synthesized in the skin from sun exposure to UVB rays.[67] Athletes, in particular, need vitamin D for its bone and immune benefits, as well as for muscle growth/repair and cardiovascular health.[30] Vitamin D also may aid in injury recovery and neuromuscular function.[3] Without it, calcium and phosphorus absorption are limited to only 10% to 15% and 60%, respectively.[67] Athletes at higher risk for insufficient/deficient vitamin D levels are those with the following:

- Higher body fat
- A history of stress fractures or bone/joint injuries

- Signs of overtraining
- Muscle pain/weakness
- Darker complexion
- Training/competition being mainly indoors or during nonpeak UVB hours
- Those living at the 35th parallel of latitude or north due to weakened sun rays[3]

Additionally, female athletes with dietary restrictions or eating disorders may be at higher risk for deficiency/insufficiency.

The Institute of Medicine (IOM) considers vitamin D levels greater than 20 ng/mL *sufficient* and levels greater than 40 ng/mL *optimal*.[30,68] Scientists disagree on these levels, and many think lower limits should be increased. Current research is equivocal on the impact of vitamin D on performance partly due to these disagreements on the definition of vitamin D deficiency; however, *deficiencies* have been found to diminish muscle repair.[69] Levels greater than 30 ng/mL protect the musculoskeletal system, and ≥40 ng/mL support stress fracture prevention, although dosages exceeding 50 ng/mL do not appear to provide additional sports health benefits.[69]

Tomlinson and colleagues[70] found that vitamin D3 supplementation improved upper and lower limb strength. Cannell and colleagues[71] discovered improvements in peak athletic performance in vitamin D–deficient athletes with supplementation of 50 ng/mL. In a blinded intervention, female naval recruits reported fewer stress fractures with supplementation of 800 IU vitamin D and 2000 mg calcium.[67] Additionally, a 2006 study showed an increased fracture risk when vitamin D intake was less than 30 ng/mL.[67] Lewis and colleagues[72] also reported that 77% of injuries in swimmers and divers coincided with decreases in 25-hydroxyvitamin D (25[OH]D), and suggested that 4000 IU may be an inexpensive method for increasing levels and protecting bone health, although larger studies are needed.

Because of the limited amount available in food, vitamin D supplementation may be recommended. The IOM recommends 400 to 600 IU per day for children and adults (0–70 years old), and 800 IU per day for older adults (>70 years), whereas the Endocrine Society recommends 400 to 1000 IU per day for infants, 600 to 1000 IU per day in children (1–18 years old), and 1500 to 2000 IU per day in adults.[68] The upper limit is between 2500 and 10,000 IU per day depending on age and recommending organization (IOM vs Endocrine Society).[67] High-dose supplementation is not recommended, as recent evidence shows possible negative effects on the vitamin D endocrine pathway and the kidneys.[3]

Current research reported that 80% of athletes with deficient or insufficient 25(OH)D may restore levels back to optimum with only 3 months of supplementation at a level of 2200 IU daily.[73] Similarly, other studies suggest the need for 3 to 5 months of supplementation to significantly raise vitamin D levels.[74] A 1-μg dose (40 IU) of vitamin D would increase 25(OH)D by 0.28 to 0.8 ng/mL in subjects with 25(OH)D levels less than 30 ng/mL at baseline.[75,76] In groups in which participants were deemed deficient in vitamin D, an added 10 μg daily was found to be beneficial in raising 25(OH)D levels.[76]

Recent evidence on female distance runners in the southeastern United States indicated that most subjects have sufficient levels of vitamin D.[77] Two factors contributed to adequate levels: locations at the latitude of 30.4° North and outdoor training. Although additional supporting data are needed, the investigators suggest that supplementation is unnecessary for most outdoor female athletes in this group. However, serum measurements may prove beneficial to identify the few athletes who still present with insufficient levels despite training in these locations.[77] Conversely, a study on NCAA athletes (66% female athletes) in the south (latitudes 35.3–36.12°N) showed that 23% were *insufficient* (20–30 ng/mL) in vitamin D and 9% were *deficient* (<20 ng/mL).[78] Those with lower vitamin D status showed reduced performance scores.

Additionally, almost 70% of athletes in another recent study (47% female athletes) also showed deficient or insufficient 25(OH)D levels, and previous research indicated that many athletes displayed serum concentrations ranging from 4 to 32 ng/mL.[67,73] Other sport-specific research reported low vitamin D as well, with 39.2% of swimmers and 80.0% of collegiate female runners failing to meet vitamin D recommendations.[7,47] Most data indicate that vitamin D insufficiency is prevalent in 33% to 42% of female athletes,[79] although the recent data by Wentz and colleagues[77] contradict this research. Therefore, regular serum measurements of athletes are recommended to continue to provide evidence that female athletes are at a higher risk than nonathletes for low serum 25(OH)D levels. Although research is limited on the effect of vitamin D on performance, some data support its importance, and the critical role that vitamin D plays in maintaining the health of an athlete. Therefore, athletes should focus on maintaining optimal 25(OH)D levels. More female-specific research is needed to determine optimum and safe supplementation levels for increasing serum 25(OH)D and its effect on performance, as availability of sufficient vitamin D in foods is limited.

Zinc

Zinc is a mineral important in muscle function and metabolic processes, resulting in decreased endurance when levels are low.[80] True zinc deficiency is rare, although individuals with anorexia nervosa (AN) are at risk.[61] Collegiate and adolescent female athletes report low zinc intake most likely due to losses through skin, sweat, and skeletal muscle breakdown.[61,80] Additionally, athletes with low EA and vegan/vegetarian athletes are more vulnerable due to low content and bioavailability in plant foods.[61] Although female athletes lose less zinc than males, they may be at higher risk due to lower dietary intakes.[80] **Table 4** provides an overview of the RDA for zinc in females.

Enhancing zinc levels is best achieved through food, as supplemental zinc may affect the absorption of iron and copper, and decrease HDL levels. Foods high in iron also provide a substantial source of zinc. Supplementation is recommended only under medical supervision and when deficiency has been found.[61] However, Eskici and colleagues[80] recently found that 4 weeks of zinc supplementation (220 mg/d) in female athletes did not change urinary excretion of magnesium, calcium, copper, and phosphorus. Careful monitoring of the duration and dosage of supplementation is important, as well as measured baseline levels before supplementation, which this study did not provide.[80] These conflicting data highlight the need for additional research on the safety and benefits of zinc supplementation in female athletes.

Calcium

Calcium is a mineral essential to female athletes for structural bone health, but also for its role in blood clotting, muscle contractions, nerve transmission, protein utilization,

Table 4	
Recommended dietary allowance for zinc: females	
Years of Age	**mg/d**
9 to >70	8
Pregnant	11
Lactating	12

Data from Hinton P. Trace minerals of concern for female athletes: iron and zinc. In: Beals K, editor. Nutrition and the female athlete; 2013. p. 96.

and cellular communication.[67] The regulation of serum calcium is controlled by para-thyroid hormone, calcitonin, and vitamin D, reinforcing the importance of optimal vitamin D intake.[67] It has been found that 72% to 90% of all females fail to meet the 1997 Adequate Intake (AI) level of calcium.[67] Barrack and colleagues[81] reported that 85% of female runners with increased bone turnover failed to meet the AI for cal-cium. Females with delayed menarche are at increased risk for low bone mineral den-sity (BMD) due to the role of estrogen in movement of calcium into the bone during bone accrual.[67] When calcium levels are sufficient, bone injuries in women appear to decrease. As discussed previously, female naval recruits developed fewer stress fractures when supplemented with 2000 mg calcium.[82] See **Table 5** for the current RDA levels for calcium in females.

It is estimated that excessive supplementation of calcium (>1500 mg/d in adoles-cents and >1100 mg/d in adults) provides no additional benefit in bone health.[67] This maximum threshold may be higher for athletes exhibiting restricted EI or men-strual dysfunction, as well as endurance athletes, who lose calcium in sweat and urine.[3,83] The current recommendation for athletes with disordered eating, amenor-rhea, or early risk for osteoporosis is 1500 mg/d of calcium.[84] A recent study concluded that the exercise-induced rise in markers of bone resorption is decreased with a high-calcium (~1350 mg) meal consumed approximately 90 minutes before prolonged, high-intensity cycling.[85] Ideally, calcium should be consumed primarily through diet, as recent evidence suggests a possible link between supplemental cal-cium intakes (as low as 500 mg) and adverse cardiovascular and kidney events.[64,86] It is also important to note that the positive effects of supplemental calcium on BMD are negligible soon after cessation of the supplement.[83]

Most research claims that calcium intake in athletes is lacking. Some data indicated that 50% of adolescent female swimmers exhibited deficient calcium intakes, although they were higher than controls.[7] The female swimmers had lower body mass index scores and a significant decrease in bone z-scores.[7] Nutrition may have played a significant role in these values, with inadequate EI in 48% of swimmers, low phosphorus intake in both groups (~33%), and insufficient calcium intake in all subjects.[7] Other studies also showed that calcium intake in 100% of adolescent fe-male athletes studied were below AI levels, and only 45% of female endurance ath-letes met the RDA for calcium.[8,65] Inadequate calcium intake is associated with disordered eating, restricted EI, and avoidance of dairy/calcium-rich foods.[3]

Magnesium
The mineral magnesium is critical for female athletes to support metabolic processes, energy production, oxygen uptake, and electrolyte balance, as well as cardiovascular, neuromuscular, immune, and hormonal functions.[84,87] Dietary magnesium is often inadequate in athletes, particularly vegetarians, vegans, or those with restricted

Table 5	
Recommended dietary allowance for calcium: females	
Years of Age	**mg/d**
9–18	1300
19–50	1000
51 to >70	1200

Data from Spence K. Nutrients needed for optimal bone health in the female athlete. In: Beals K, editor. Nutrition and the female athlete; 2013. p. 124.

El.[84] Additionally, exercise increases magnesium requirements through accelerated losses via sweat and urine.[88] Some scientists propose that magnesium intake by athletes should be 10% to 20% higher than current recommendations for the general public.[87]

Low magnesium intake increases the oxygen cost of exercise, which may impair endurance performance.[84] Depletion also amplifies neuromuscular excitability due to increased calcium retention in the muscle.[87,89] Levels of magnesium intake have been found to predict swim times in female athletes as well as affect jump execution in volleyball athletes.[87] Appropriate levels also have been associated with the prevention of age-related decline in work output in active older women.[90] However, some studies show no effect of magnesium supplementation on performance.[90]

The RDA for magnesium in females is 310 to 320 mg/d, although it is estimated that only approximately 70% of women meet recommended levels.[89,90] Magnesium deficiency is considered less than 220 mg/d for female athletes.[87] Research shows that most female athletes across a variety of sports report low intakes, with weight-class sports at highest risk due to restricted El.[84,90]

A severe magnesium deficiency, although rare in athletes, may cause muscle weakness, muscle cramps, neuromuscular dysfunction, and immunosuppression.[87] It is commonly thought that magnesium supplementation may relieve muscle cramps, yet very few studies support this. Those that did suggested hypomagnesemia as the root cause of the cramps. Further investigation clarifying the association between magnesium and cramping are needed and could prove extremely beneficial for the many athletes who suffer from cramping during competition.[87] Magnesium appears to impart other health benefits in addition. Supplementation in female athletes with low serum magnesium was found to improve muscular responses to training.[89] It may also assist with bone homeostasis, antioxidant defense, DNA preservation, and cell membrane stabilization[88,90,91] However, magnesium supplementation appears to only provide beneficial effects in athletes whose levels are deficient.[87]

Current research supports a need for higher magnesium intakes in female athletes, although stronger studies are necessary to rule out any confounding variables from lack of baseline measures, less accurate measurement methods (serum or plasma magnesium), and gender differences.

B vitamins

Research indicates that athletes may have a higher requirement for the B vitamins due to increased metabolic processing, biochemical adaptations in tissue, increased need for repair/maintenance of large quantities of lean tissue, and accelerated turnover in sweat, urine, and feces.[84,92] Folate and vitamin B12 (cobalamin) are important in red blood cell (RBC) formation and cellular repair.[84] The other B vitamins (thiamin, riboflavin, niacin, pyridoxine, pantothenic acid, and biotin) are necessary as coenzymes in metabolism.[84] Supplementation with most of the B vitamins offers no added benefit when an athlete's dietary intake provides optimal amounts. Although evidence shows that most athletes consume most B vitamins in adequate levels, some research reports that female endurance athletes are more likely to consume less than the RDA of B vitamins, especially vegetarians (or those with low beef, dairy, and poultry intakes) and those with eating disorders or restricted El.[65] Further studies are needed in female athletes specifically. The RDA and AI levels for the B vitamins can be found in **Table 6**. The B vitamins with the most pertinent data for athletes are discussed in more detail in the following paragraphs.

Riboflavin (vitamin B2) needs are higher for female athletes than for sedentary women, with requirements increasing to as much as 2 mg/d.[92]

Table 6			
B vitamins for females			
Recommended Dietary Allowance		**Adequate Intake**	
Folate, μg/d	400	Pantothenic Acid, mg/d	5
Pregnancy	600	Biotin, μg/d	30
Lactation	500	Choline, μg/d	425
Vitamin B12, μg/d	2.4		
Thiamin, mg/d	1.1		
Riboflavin, mg/d	1.1		
Niacin, mg/d	14		
Vitamin B6, mg/d	1.3		

Data from Burke L, Dziedzic C. Carbohydrate requirements for the female athlete. In: Beals K, editor. Nutrition and the female athlete; 2013. p. 29.

Niacin (vitamin B3) supplementation may have detrimental effects on performance, preventing the typical rise in free fatty acids (FFAs) seen with activity.[92] Although validation is needed in humans, recent data in mice has shown that supplementation with nicotinamide riboside (a pyridine-nucleoside form of niacin) may increase skeletal muscle mitochondrial biogenesis, which could ultimately assist with EA.[30]

Pyridoxine (vitamin B6) plays a role in the synthesis of niacin, as well as amino acid metabolism and glycogen breakdown.[92] Exercise may influence vitamin B6 metabolism, increasing pyridoxal 5-phosphate (the active form of B6), and the turnover of B6 within the body.[92] Supplementation does not improve performance and lowers FFA concentration in exercising females.[92]

Folate is known mostly for its role in preventing neural tube defects (NTDs) in newborns.[92] As many female athletes are in their child-bearing years, they have increased requirements for folate. Maintenance of optimal folate levels is imperative to maintain during these years, as NTDs form in the 4 weeks after conception, when many women do not realize that they are pregnant.[93] Folate serves other additional roles in the body, such as RBC formation, DNA synthesis, and cellular repair/maintenance.[92]

Most research suggests that female athletes are at risk for inadequate folate levels due to poor dietary intake.[92] In military studies, folate status declined in females during a 12-day training course, and a significant number of cadets did not meet the RDA.[93] Very few studies have analyzed folate's role in athletic performance, although one study revealed that even with high-dose folate supplementation and increased serum levels, there was no performance improvement in female marathoners.[92]

Cobalamin, or *vitamin B12*, is essential for converting folate into its active form, and thus plays its own role in RBC formation, tissue repair/maintenance, DNA synthesis, and fatty acid metabolism.[92] Some research states that the risk for poor vitamin B12 status in athletes is low, whereas others report female athletes exhibit decreased dietary intakes. Vegetarian/vegan female athletes and those with low EA are also at a higher risk for insufficient B12.[3,92] The existing performance data show that supplementation has no notable benefit in male athletes consuming a well-balanced diet; female athletes were not studied.[92] If severe deficiency of vitamin B12 and/or folate results in anemia, endurance performance may decline.[84]

Antioxidants

Antioxidants are nutrients that protect against oxidative stress. Although exercise increases oxidative damage, the body's response is enhanced functioning of its endogenous antioxidant systems.[3] Therefore, athletes may not benefit from added antioxidant supplementation, as research suggests that nondietary sources do not enhance performance. Some studies have also shown that doses above "tolerable upper-intake levels" become pro-oxidative in training. Consequently, choosing a diet high in antioxidant-rich foods is safer than supplementing.[3] Antioxidants are heterogeneous and each works in a different way; therefore, variety in the diet is important.[30] Athletes at highest risk for poor antioxidant status are those with low EA, and those following a low-fat diet or a diet low in fruits, vegetables, and whole grains.[3] Further research in female athletes is needed.

Vitamin E has been shown to have some beneficial effects with supplementation, reducing lipid peroxidation, attenuating exercise-induced DNA damage, and possibly enhancing postexercise recovery.[84] More research is needed to investigate the possible negative effects of supplementation, and to provide supporting evidence on its safety.

Vitamin C does not have an ergogenic effect on performance when dietary intake is at an optimal level. However, vitamin C needs increase with prolonged activity; therefore, athletes must ensure 100 to 1000 mg daily with habitual prolonged, strenuous exercise.[84]

Selenium is an antioxidant found in abundance in muscle tissue, which makes its role significant in an athlete's diet. Research is equivocal on whether athletes need more than the general public, and supplementation has not yet proven to enhance performance. However, athletes at increased risk for poor antioxidant status may benefit from additional selenium, as deficiency is known to cause muscle tiredness and weakened muscle concentrations in athletes.[80] Supplementation effects in humans have not been thoroughly studied, although both zinc and selenium in exercising rats prevented the oxidative stress caused by exercise.[80]

Hydration

Optimal fluid and electrolyte balance is imperative in athletic performance. Muscular contractions and metabolic heat generation from exercise increase body temperature and, thus, fluid requirements.[3] Although there is disagreement, most research supports that losing greater than 2% of one's BW in sweat may compromise cognitive function and aerobic exercise in the heat. A loss of 3% to 5% of BW may negatively affect aerobic and anaerobic, high-intensity exercise in a cool environment, as well as skill performance in hot/humid conditions.[3,94] Typical sweat rates are approximately 0.3 to 2.4 L/h, which vary based on humidity, ambient temperature, fitness level, altitude, heat acclimatization, BW, genetics, metabolic efficiency, and exercise intensity and duration.[3,84] Numerous studies have found that many athletes (>30%) begin exercise in a dehydrated state based on urine specific gravity (USG), only to become more dehydrated at the conclusion of activity (>43% of athletes studied).[95–97]

Research shows that the regulation of fluid-electrolyte balance differs in women compared with men. Women have lower sweat rates, lower plasma volumes, and lower potassium and sodium sweat concentrations.[98] Due to smaller body size and greater body surface area–to-BW ratio, women produce 18% to 34% less sweat per hour than men during exercise.[99] Sweat rates in females are even lower in hot, wet environments due to the greater surface area–to-BW ratio, and thus a greater skin area available for evaporative sweating. This allows female athletes to maintain their core temperature and retain a thermoregulatory advantage over men.[98] Additionally, women have been found to consume more fluids relative to their body size. Moreover, some of this difference may be attributed in part to fluctuations in hormonal levels within the menstrual cycle.[99] Body water may increase by 2 L from the follicular to the luteal phase.[99] Higher estrogen levels during the luteal phase lower a female's thermoregulatory threshold due to plasma volume expansion.[98] Although beneficial in some cases, faster onset of sweating at a lower core temperature may increase body water losses more quickly, increasing risk for dehydration.[98] Women also have lower arginine vasopressin concentration (the hormone that regulates renal free water), allowing for an increase in sodium and fluid retention, and a lower urine osmolality.[99] However, most research indicates that the differences caused by hormonal fluctuations in women do not appear to affect performance, fluid regulation, or health risks during exercise.[98] As women become more trained, the sex differences in hydration status between men and women decrease, although continued research on gender differences is still lacking and would provide further clarification.

Current American College of Sports Medicine guidelines recommend that fluid and sodium needs be based on individual measurement of fluid and sodium losses, which would support sex-specific parameters. The guidelines also can be adapted to women by adjusting for BW.[100] **Box 1** provides the most recent guidelines for hydration needs surrounding exercise.

There is not an optimal, error-free way to track hydration, although daily morning BW changes (postvoid) may provide an easy, quick status for athletes who are in energy balance.[3] More specific methods are USG and urinary osmolality, which measure urinary solute concentration.[3] Recent data, however, show low specificity in the use of USG in NCAA athletes, suggesting caution be taken when using this as a field measure.[101] More recent data support the use of bioelectrical impedance spectroscopy for assessing the hydration status of elite athletes,[102] although additional research is needed.

Hyponatremia

Hyponatremia is defined as blood sodium levels less than 135 mmol/L, often caused by overdrinking of water, excess sodium losses without sufficient replacement, and

---

Box 1
Fluid needs

Before Exercise (2–4 hours prior)

- Consume 5 to 10 mL/kg body weight (BW).
  - Include sodium to assist with fluid retention.

During Exercise

- 0.4 to 0.8 L/h customized to athlete's tolerance and experience.
- Cold and flavored beverages may increase palatability.
- Carbohydrate and sodium may enhance fluid/electrolyte balance.
- Carbohydrate concentrations of less than 8% and hypotonic fluid decrease gastric emptying.

After Exercise

- Consume normal meals and fluids if there is adequate time to rehydrate.
- Rapid and complete rehydration: consume 1.25 to 1.5 L for every 1 kg BW lost.
- Increase intake of sodium-rich foods.
- Sweat losses and obligatory urine losses continue during postexercise. Stay diligent.

Data from Thomas DT, Erdman KA, Burke LM. American College of Sports Medicine joint position statement. Nutrition and athletic performance. Med Sci Sports Exerc 2016;48(3):543–68.

excess sweat and urinary losses.[3] Women are at a higher risk because of smaller body size, lower sweat rates, excess fluid ingestion, and longer competition times.[98] Risk for hyponatremia is even greater during the luteal phase of the menstrual cycle, when estradiol is higher and free water retention is increased.[98]

On average, sweat contains about 1 g/L of sodium.[84] Athletes with high sweat rates (>1.2 L/h) are also at a higher risk for hyponatremia and therefore are recommended to consume sodium during exercise. Sodium also should be consumed during activity lasting longer than 2 hours. Although thirst often can be a fair indicator of the need for hydration, older athletes and individual differences make this an unreliable method for some.[3]

Although research implies that the hormonal variations in women do not alter fluid or electrolyte needs enough to require women to change their hydration routines, further research is needed to investigate this and the effects of hyponatremia.[98]

Other Nutritional Issues

Runner's gut, gut ischemia, and fermentable oligosaccharides, disaccharides, monosaccharides, and polyols

Runners and other athletes often suffer from GI issues commonly referred to as "runner's gut." Multiple factors affect its presence: ischemic, mechanical, and nutritional.[21] The effects of nutritional factors on the GI tract during exercise have limited data, but some are discussed here. For a more comprehensive discussion, the reader is referred to the article on Gastrointestinal Concerns of the Female Athlete, by Barry Kent Diduch's article, "Gastrointestinal Conditions in the Female Athlete," in this issue.

When GI function is compromised, nausea, vomiting, diarrhea, bloody stools, and abdominal angina may affect the athlete's performance.[103] Splanchnic hypoperfusion resulting in a relative hypoxic environment is the main mechanism causing symptoms, which is experienced by 25% to 70% of endurance athletes.[103] This decreased blood flow to the gut can lead to GI ischemia.[21] On reperfusion, the damaged GI mucosa loses some of its gut barrier effectiveness. This results in increased permeability, allowing for bacterial translocation and generation of endotoxins, resulting in distress.

It is recommended that high protein, fiber, and fat intake be avoided within 2 to 3 hours of activity due to slow digestibility.[103] Small amounts of easily digestible food are best before and during exercise, making MTCs an ideal choice for maintaining energy stores.[103] However, ingestion of carbohydrates in higher temperatures may delay gastric emptying and cause fluid shifts, leading to diarrhea.[21] Because the intestinal absorption rate of glucose is 1.0 to 1.2 g/min, intakes lower than 1.2 g/min are recommended. Adequate hydration is also essential to prevent systemic hypovolemia and maintain splanchnic perfusion during exercise.[103] Carbohydrate concentrations ≤8% in beverages are best to reduce the occurrence of diarrhea associated with high osmolar fluids.[21] After exercise, consuming lipids may decrease intestinal inflammation, leading to improved GI function and splanchnic blood flow, and reduce the symptoms commonly associated with endotoxemia after intense activity.[103]

In attempts to prevent "runner's gut," tactics aiming to supplement with products that increase nitric oxide (NO) are popular. NO is an effective vasodilator, thus thought to help with the relative problems caused by hypoperfusion. It is hypothesized that supplementation with any of the many precursors leading to the production of NO will increase its availability and prove helpful to the body. These precursors include *arginine* (direct precursor to NO), *citrulline* (precursor to arginine), and *glutamine* (precursor to citrulline). Each has varying degrees of evidence to support its effectiveness with supplementation. *Nitrate*, found in food and beetroot supplements, is reduced to nitrite and NO. It may be an ideal option for preventing exercise-associated GI issues through increased gastric blood flow.[103] It has also been shown to increase exercise tolerance, improve time-trial performance, and decrease oxidative stress.[103] Any supplements should be used with caution, as most are not independently tested for contaminants and efficacy, and many are unnecessary if a well-balanced diet is maintained.

Some commonly used substances, such as caffeine and NSAIDs, may infer risk to the GI system in the unknowing athlete. High-dose caffeine use is widespread among athletes, causing increased GI distress. Decreasing dosages to 3 mg/kg show some benefit in effectively reducing symptoms.[21] NSAID use also increases risk of upper GI issues, and can result in intestinal injury and mucosal bleeding.[21,103] NSAIDs reduce blood flow to the upper GI tract and may interfere with NO production, inducing vasoconstriction when intestinal inflammation is present.[103]

FODMAPs (fermentable oligosaccharides, disaccharides, monosaccharides, and polyols) are poorly absorbed, short-chain carbohydrates found in various fruits and vegetables, wheat, onions, sorbitol, and some dairy products.[21] High FODMAP intake has been shown to draw water into the intestine and cause fermentation, generating gas and diarrhea. Scientists suggest that the repetitive stress and gut injury induced by exercise places added risk of GI symptoms from FODMAPs on athletes compared with their nonactive counterparts.[21] Some athletes (almost 65% of them female) had fewer GI symptoms with FODMAPs elimination.[21] A low FODMAPs diet is primarily used in those with irritable bowel disease (IBD), and has been proven effective in treating GI symptoms (82% of the patients were female).[104] Female athletes may be at greater risk for IBD and other GI issues compared with both female nonathletes and all males due to the higher prevalence of IBD in women in addition to the stress of exercise on the gut.[104] However, more research is needed to evaluate the effect of each of the nutritional strategies discussed on GI issues in female athletes, including additional studies of the effects of dehydration, the long-term use of supplements, and low FODMAPs diets.

Celiac disease
Little research has been done on CD in athletes. CD may cause bone loss in adults, which poses an increased risk of injury to female athletes, especially those with low EA or amenorrhea.[105] Endurance athletes with CD may be at a higher risk for performance issues due to the challenges of consuming enough energy from gluten-free (GF) foods during heavy training.[106] There has been a rise in GF diet use in athletes due to the perceived performance and GI benefits. Forty percent of nonceliac endurance cyclists studied by Lis and colleagues[107] followed a GF diet; however, no significant differences were found in GI symptoms, inflammatory markers, indicators of intestinal injury, or well-being. It is important to note that following a GF diet when medically unnecessary and without proper knowledge may lead to inadequate intake of fiber, iron, B vitamins, and reduced beneficial gut bacteria.[107] Additionally, controlling for FODMAP intake in celiac research is important to ensure accurate outcomes. In subjects following a GF diet, improvement of symptoms was higher in those also following a low-FODMAP diet.[107]

Microbiome and eating disorders
New research is beginning to investigate the gut-brain axis and its influence on AN outcomes. Evidence continues to indicate that the gut microbiome interacts with the central nervous system, and may influence weight regulation and psychopathology.[108] Starvation and long-term dieting alter the makeup of the gut microbiome

and the growth of bacterial species, causing "leaky gut" symptoms commonly seen in those with AN.[108] Females with AN exhibited reduced diversity of bacteria in the gut microbiome and higher levels of specific bacterial groups that are significantly associated with depression scores and eating disorder psychopathology.[108] Although prevalence numbers for eating disorders in female athletes vary from 8% to 47%, the presence of disordered eating issues in the athletic population makes this an important and innovative area of research.[109]

Research also indicates that Western diets (animal protein, sugar, and fat) and non-Western diets (plant-derived carbohydrates) alter the gut microbiome, with quick responses to acute modifications in macronutrient intake occurring within 3 to 4 days of such dietary changes.[108] Subjects consuming an animal-based diet presented with higher levels of the bacteria known to have a high bile resistance, as well as an increased risk for development of IBD.[108] This may be important in anorexic athletes, as changing from their typical plant-based, high-fiber diet to the high-calorie, high-fat, high-carbohydrate diet commonly seen in recovery may increase the growth of inflammatory gut bacteria. However, more human data are needed to support these theories.

Prebiotics and probiotics also are imperative in the health of the microbiome. *Prebiotics* are the "nondigestible food ingredients that induce the growth of microorganisms that contribute to the well-being of their host,"[108] such as fructans, milk oligosaccharides, pectins, and glucans. Prebiotics improve the gut microbiome, reducing inflammation, enhancing cognitive function, and lessening depressive or anxious states.[108] *Probiotics* are "living component[s] of the microbiota administered to humans or animals that are associated with health benefits for the host."[108] It is thought that probiotics reduce intestinal permeability, reverse neuropsychological deficits found from repeat antibiotic use, and in mice, reduce depressive and anxiety-like behavior.[108] Other effects of probiotics important to athletes include decreased upper respiratory tract infections, reduced immunosuppression, and enhanced absorption of nutrients.[110] Only 1 study directly analyzed the ergogenic effects of probiotics (in hotter temperatures) in athletes, showing a moderate increase in time to exhaustion, and decreased gut permeability and GI distress in runners.[110] Athletes using probiotics should begin use at least 14 days before travel or competition to allow for colonization of bacterial species in the gut, and to ensure any common, mild side effects (flatulence, gut pain) are no longer present.[110] Again, care should be taken when choosing a brand of supplements to ensure highest quality and no contamination. Continued research on prebiotics and probiotics is important to refine understanding of beneficial strains, mechanisms, dose-response, effects on performance, and specific effects on the female athlete.[110]

Supplements

Supplements are a broad topic with much controversy and few have good scientific backing. Athletes should remain cautious about the use of supplements unless they can find independently drug-tested products and have a clear rationale for their use in addition to an otherwise well-balanced diet.[30] Most commercial supplements are not safe, not effective, or do not provide optimal, research-based doses of the compound being marketed. Most supplement research has been done in male athletes, with little gender-specific research on women. It is outside the scope of this article to discuss supplements in detail. The supplements with the most scientific research are examined briefly in the following paragraphs, in addition to nitrates/beetroot juice, prebiotics/probiotics, antioxidants, vitamin D, and other micronutrients (when levels are deficient), which were reviewed earlier in the article.

Caffeine is a modifier of muscle contractility, and is most widely known for its benefit in reducing the perception of effort, fatigue, or pain during exercise.[30] The use of caffeine can enhance training outcomes, allowing athletes to train at higher intensities or for longer durations. The most common recommended dose is 3 mg/kg, although negative side effects are possible. Caution must be taken in the implementation of caffeine, as dangerous health outcomes may occur when mixed with other stimulants or consumed at high doses.[30] There is also evolving research showing individual variation in response to caffeine use.[30]

Creatine is "an amino acid–derived metabolite found predominantly in skeletal muscle from both endogenous synthesis and dietary intake (meat)."[30] The goal of creatine supplementation is to optimize muscle stores. Creatine monohydrate is the most effective form, coingested with carbohydrates.[30] Supplementation may increase generation of ATP for high-intensity sports or intense training.[30] Current research disputes concerns of decreased thermoregulation and muscle damage.[30] Typical recommended dosages are 2 to 5 g/d.[111] Some research supports a loading phase of 20 g/d for 1 week; however, the loading phase is unnecessary if the athlete has at least a month to achieve body composition goals. Dosages of 3 g/d of creatine for 28 days have been found to produce the same outcomes as the 1-week load.[111]

Omega-3 polyunsaturated fatty acids (PUFAs) include eicosapentaenoic acid, docosahexaenoic acid, and more recently docosapentaenoic acid. These are widely known for their role in cardiovascular health, and may further benefit the athlete with an impact on inflammation, skeletal muscle metabolism, glucose homeostasis, and brain health. Research is limited regarding the performance benefits of omega-3 PUFAs, but there are some human data showing a role in intrinsic anabolic/anticatabolic properties in maintaining protein balance.[112] Studies are needed to assess the effect of omega-3 PUFAs on long-term muscle outcomes. Omega-3 PUFAs also have been shown to improve glucose homeostasis and fatty acid insulin resistance.[112] One exercise study reported a reduction in glucose flux and an increase in fat oxidation.[112] Although there is limited human research, the available data appear promising for the role of omega-3 PUFAs in concussion prevention and recovery. Omega-3 PUFAs provide brain structure, support brain signaling, decrease acute axon loss, cut inflammation in the brain, lessen oxidative stress, and reduce glutamate cytotoxicity.[113] Dosage recommendations vary from 1500 to 18,000 mg, but lower doses have been proven safe for maintenance and prevention.[112]

Beta-alanine is the rate-limiting precursor to carnosine synthesis, with research supporting its intracellular buffering capacity through increased muscle carnosine.[30] It has been found to improve performance in high-intensity sports and enhance exercise training by reducing acid-base disturbances.[3] The optimal loading protocol needs more scientific backing; however, some data support increased beta-alanine buffering by 50% to 85% with intakes of 3 to 6 g/d for 4 to 12 weeks.[30] Beta-alanine can be found naturally in meats.

SUMMARY

The female athlete has nutritional needs that may vary from those of male athletes. Although there is extensive research on the macronutrient, micronutrient, and fluid needs of athletes, much of these data have been completed in male subjects. Female athletes are at higher risk for GI issues and eating disorders, so careful attention to these areas also is pertinent. Care must be taken when providing nutritional recommendations to athletes, as consideration of the intensity, duration, phase of training, and sport, as well as their body size and gender is important.

REFERENCES

1. Nattiv A, Loucks AB, Manore MM, et al. American College of Sports Medicine position stand. The female triad. Med Sci Sports Exerc 2007;39(10):1867–82.
2. Beals K. Energy availability, health, and performance in the female athlete. In: Beals, K, editor. Nutrition and the female athlete. Boca Raton, London, New York: CRC Press; 2013.
3. Thomas DT, Erdman KA, Burke LM. American College of Sports Medicine Joint Position Statement. Nutrition and athletic performance. Med Sci Sports Exerc 2016;48(3):543–68.
4. Slater J, McLay-Cooke R, Brown R, et al. Female recreational exercisers at risk for low energy availability. Int J Sport Nutr Exerc Metab 2016;26(5):421–7.
5. Koutedakis Y, Jamurtas A. The dancer as a performing athlete: physiological considerations. Sports Med 2004;34(10):651–61.
6. Gibson JC, Stuart-Hill L, Martin S, et al. Nutrition status of junior elite Canadian female soccer athletes. Int J Sport Nutr Exerc Metab 2011;21(6):507–14.
7. Lee N, Kim J. A review of the effect of swim training and nutrition on bone mineral density in female athletes. J Exerc Nutrition Biochem 2015;19(4):273–9.
8. Coutinho LA, Porto CP, Pierucci AP. Critical evaluation of food intake and energy balance in young modern pentathlon athletes: a cross-sectional study. J Int Soc Sports Nutr 2016;13:15.
9. Vanheest JL, Rodgers CD, Mahoney CE, et al. Ovarian suppression impairs sport performance in junior elite female swimmers. Med Sci Sports Exerc 2014;46(1):156–66.
10. Hand TM, Howe S, Ciadella-Kam L, et al. A pilot study: dietary energy density is similar between active women with and without exercise-associated menstrual dysfunction. Nutrients 2016;8(4):230.
11. Reed JL, Bowell JL, Hill BR, et al. Exercising women with menstrual disturbances consume low energy dense foods and beverages. Appl Physiol Nutr Metab 2011;36(3):382–94.
12. Burke L, Hawley J, Wong S, et al. Carbohydrates for training and competition. J Sports Sci 2011;29:S17–27.
13. Burke L, Kiens B, Ivy J. Carbohydrates and fat for training and recovery. J Sports Sci 2004;22(1):15–30.
14. Burke L, Dziedzic C. Carbohydrate requirements for the female athlete. In: Beals K, editor. Nutrition and the female athlete. 2013.
15. Burke LM, Cox GR, Culmmings NK, et al. Guidelines for daily carbohydrate intake: do athletes achieve them? Sports Med 2001;31:267–99.
16. Tarnopolsky M, Zawada C, Richmond L, et al. Gender differences in carbohydrate loading are related to energy intake. J Appl Physiol (1985) 2001;91(1):225–30.
17. Masson G, Lamarche B. Many non-elite multisport endurance athletes do not meet sports nutrition recommendations for carbohydrates. Appl Physiol Nutr Metab 2016;41(7):728–34.
18. Paul DR, Mulroy SM, Horner JA, et al. Carbohydrate-loading during the follicular phase of the menstrual cycle: effects on muscle glycogen and exercise performance. Int J Sport Nutr Exerc Metab 2001;11(4):430–41.
19. Bam J, Noakes T, Juritz J, et al. Could women outrun men in ultramarathon races? Med Sci Sports Exerc 1997;29(2):244–7.
20. Coyle E. Fluid and fuel intake during exercise. J Sports Sci 2004;22(1):39–55.

21. de Oliveira EP. Runner's diarrhea: what is it, what causes it, and how can it be prevented? Curr Opin Gastroenterol 2017;33(1):41–6.
22. Ormsbee MJ, Gorman KA, Miller EA, et al. Nighttime feeding likely alters morning metabolism but not exercise performance in female athletes. Appl Physiol Nutr Metab 2016;41(7):719–27.
23. Roy BD, Luttmer K, Bosman MJ, et al. The influence of post-exercise macronutrient intake on energy balance and protein metabolism in active females participating in endurance endurance training. Int J Sport Nutr Exerc Metab 2002;12(2):172–88.
24. Betts JA, Williams C. Short-term recovery from prolonged exercise: exploring the potential for protein ingestion to accentuate the benefits of carbohydrate supplements. Sports Med 2010;40(11):941–59.
25. Bartlett JD, Hawley JA, Morton JP. Carbohydrate availability and exercise training adaptation: too much of a good thing? Eur J Sport Sci 2015;15(1):3–12.
26. Burke LM. Fueling strategies to optimize performance: training high or training low? Scand J Med Sci Sports 2010;20(Suppl 2):48–58.
27. Cox GR, Clark SA, Cox AJ, et al. Daily training with high carbohydrate availability increases exogenous carbohydrate oxidation during endurance cycling. J Appl Physiol (1985) 2010;109(1):126–34.
28. Howarth KR, Phillips SM, Macdonald MJ, et al. Effect of glycogen availability on human skeletal muscle protein turnover during exercise and recovery. J Appl Physiol (1985) 2010;109:431–8.
29. Taylor C, Bartlett JD, van de Graaf CS, et al. Protein ingestion does not impair exercise-induced AMPK signalling when in a glycogen-depleted state: implications for train-low compete-high. Eur J Appl Physiol 2013;113:1457–68.
30. Close GL, Hamilton DL, Philip A, et al. New strategies in sport nutrition to increase exercise performance. Free Radic Biol Med 2016;98:144–58.
31. Gleeson M, Nieman DC, Pedersen BK. Exercise, nutrition and immune function. J Sports Sci 2004;22(1):115–25.
32. Hausswirth C, Le Meur Y. Physiological and nutritional aspects of post-exercise recovery: specific recommendations for female athletes. Sports Med 2011;41(10):861–82.
33. Maher A, Tarnopolsky M. Substrate utilization in female athletes: implications for fuel selection and macronutrient requirements. In: Beals K, editor. Nutrition and the female athlete. 2013.
34. Sarafian D, Schutz Y, Montani JP, et al. Sex difference in substrate oxidation during low-instensity isometric exercise in young adults. Appl Physiol Nutr Metab 2016;41(9):977–84.
35. Zehnder M, Ith M, Kreis R, et al. Gender-specific usage of intramyocellular lipids and glycogen during exercise. Med Sci Sports Exerc 2005;37(9):1517–24.
36. Vogt M, Puntschart A, Howald H, et al. Effects of dietary fat on muscle substrates, metabolism, and performance in athletes. Med Sci Sports Exerc 2003;35(6):952–60.
37. Volek JS, Freidenreich DJ, Saenz C, et al. Metabolic characteristics of keto-adapted ultra-endurance runners. Metabolism 2016;65(3):100–10.
38. Urbain P, Strom L, Morawski L, et al. Impact of a 6-week non-energy-restricted ketogenic diet on physical fitness, body composition and biochemical parameters in healthy adults. Nutr Metab 2017;14:17.
39. Rodriguez N. Protein requirements for the female athlete. In: Beals K, editor. Nutrition and the female athlete. 2013.

40. Pikosky MA, Gaine PC, Martin WF, et al. Aerobic exercise training increases skeletal muscle protein turnover in healthy adults at rest. J Nutr 2006;136(2): 379–83.

41. Bolster DR, Pikosky MA, Gaine PC, et al. Dietary protein intake impacts human skeletal muscle protein fractional synthetic rates after endurance exercise. Am J Physiol Endocrinol Metab 2005;289(4):E678–83.

42. Tarnopolsky M. Protein requirements for endurance athletes. Nutrition 2004; 20(7–8):662–8.

43. Tipton KD, Witard OC. Protein requirements and recommendations for athletes: relevance of ivory tower arguments for practical recommendations. Clin Sports Med 2007;26(1):17–36.

44. Phillips SM, van Loon LJ. Dietary protein for athletes: from requirements to optimum adaptation. J Sports Sci 2011;29(Suppl 1):S29–538.

45. Wall BT, Morton JP, van Loon LJ. Strategies to maintain skeletal muscle mass in the injured athlete: nutritional considerations and exercise mimetics. Eur J Sport Sci 2015;15(1):53–62.

46. Rodriguez NR, Vislocky LM, Gaine PC. Dietary protein, endurance exercise, and human skeletal-muscle protein turnover. Curr Opin Clin Nutr Metab Care 2007; 10(1):40–5.

47. Barrack MT, Fredericson M, Kim BY, et al. Evidence of energy deficiency and low carbohydrate intake among male and female elite collegiate endurance runners. Med Sci Sports Exerc 2015;47(S2).

48. Hinton PS, Sanford TC, Davidson MM, et al. Nutrient intakes and dietary behaviors of male and female collegiate athletes. Int J Sport Nutr Exerc Metab 2004; 14(4):389–405.

49. Gillen JB, Trommelen J, Wardenaar FC, et al. Dietary protein intake and distribution patterns of well-trained Dutch athletes. Int J Sport Nutr Exerc Metab 2017; 27(2):105–14.

50. Kriengsinyos W, Wykes LJ, Goonewardene LA, et al. Phase of menstrual cycle affects lysine requirement in healthy women. Am J Physiol Endocrinol Metab 2004;287(3):E489–96.

51. Toth MJ, Sites CK, Matthews DE, et al. Ovarian suppression with gonadotropin-releasing hormone agonist reduces whole body protein turnover in women. Am J Physiol Endocrinol Metab 2006;291(3):E483–90.

52. Bailey SP, Zacher CM, Mittleman KD. Effect of menstrual cycle phase on carbohydrate supplementation during prolonged exercise to fatigue. J Appl Physiol (1985) 2000;88(2):690–7.

53. Kumar V, Atherton P, Smith K, et al. Human muscle protein synthesis and breakdown during and after exercise. J Appl Physiol (1985) 2009;106:2026–39.

54. Moore DR, Robinson MJ, Fry JL, et al. Ingested protein dose response of muscle and albumin protein synthesis after resistance exercise in young men. Am J Clin Nutr 2009;89(1):161–8.

55. Josse AR, Tang JE, Tamopolsky MA, et al. Body composition and strength changes in women with milk and resistance exercise. Med Sci Sports Exerc 2010;42(6):1122–30.

56. Areta JL, Burke LM, Ross ML, et al. Timing and distribution of protein ingestion during prolonged recovery from resistance exercise alters myofibrillar protein synthesis. J Physiol 2013;591(Pt 9):2319–31.

57. Phillips SM. A brief review of critical processes in exercise induced muscular hypertrophy. Sports Med 2014;44(Suppl 1):S71–577.

58. Arnal MA, Mosoni L, Boirie Y, et al. Protein feeding pattern does not affect protein retention in young women. J Nutr 2000;130(7):1700–4.
59. Moore DR, Churchward-Venne TA, Witard O, et al. Protein ingestion to stimulate myofibrillar protein synthesis requires greater relative protein intakes in healthy older versus younger men. J Gerontol A Biol Sci Med Sci 2015;70(1):57–62.
60. Snijders T, Res PT, Smeets JS, et al. Protein ingestion before sleep increases muscle mass and strength gains during prolonged resistance-type exercise training in healthy young men. J Nutr 2015;145:1178–84.
61. Hinton P. Trace minerals of concern for female athletes: iron and zinc. In: Beals K, editor. Nutrition and the female athlete. 2013.
62. Coates A, Mountjoy M, Burr J. Incidence of iron deficiency and iron deficient anemia in elite runners and triathletes. Clin J Sport Med 2016. [Epub ahead of print].
63. Dellavalle DM, Haas JD. Iron status is associated with endurance performance and training in female rowers. Med Sci Sports Exerc 2012;44(8):1552–9.
64. Kim BY, Nattiv A. Health considerations in female runners. Phys Med Rehabil Clin N Am 2016;27(1):151–78.
65. Baranauskas M, Stukas R, Tubelis L, et al. Nutritional habits among high-performance endurance athletes. Medicina (Kaunas) 2015;51(6):351–62.
66. Moretti D, Goede JS, Zeder C, et al. Oral iron supplements increase hepcidin and decrease iron absorption from daily or twice-daily doses in iron-depleted young women. Blood 2015;126:1981–90.
67. Spence K. Nutrients needed for optimal bone health in the female athlete. In: Beals K, editor. Nutrition and the female athlete. 2013.
68. Ogan D, Pritchett K. Vitamin D and the athlete: risks, recommendations, and benefits. Nutrients 2013;5(6):1856–68.
69. Shuler FD, Wingate MK, Moore GH, et al. Sports health benefits of vitamin D. Sports Health 2012;4(6):496–501.
70. Tomlinson PB, Joseph C, Angioi M. Effects of vitamin D supplementation on upper and lower body muscle strength levels in healthy individuals. A systematic review with meta-analysis. J Sci Med Sport 2015;18(5):575–80.
71. Cannell J, Hollis B, Sorenson M, et al. Athletic performance and vitamin D. Med Sci Sports Exerc 2009;41(5):1102–10.
72. Lewis RM, Redzic M, Thomas DT. The effects of season-long vitamin D supplementation on collegiate swimmers and divers. Int J Sport Nutr Exerc Metab 2013;23(5):431–40.
73. Backx EM, Tieland M, Maase K, et al. The impact of 1-year vitamin D supplementation on vitamin D status in athletes: a dose-response study. Eur J Clin Nutr 2016;70(9):1009–14.
74. Chao Y, Brunel L, Faris P, et al. The importance of dose, frequency, and duration of vitamin D supplementation for plasma 25-hydroxyvitamin D. Nutrients 2013;5:4067–78.
75. Heaney RP, Davies KM, Chen TC, et al. Human serum 25-hydroxycholecalciferol response to extended oral dosing with cholecalciferol. Am J Clin Nutr 2003;77:204–10.
76. Whiting SJ, Bonjour JP, Payen FD, et al. Moderate amounts of vitamin D3 in supplements are effective in raising serum 25-hydroxyvitamin D from low baseline levels in adults: a systemic review. Nutrients 2015;7(4):2311–23.
77. Wentz LM, Liu PY, Ilich JZ, et al. Female distance runners training in Southeastern United States have adequate vitamin D status. Int J Sport Nutr Exerc Metab 2016;26(5):397–403.

78. Hildebrand RA, Miller B, Warren A, et al. Compromised vitamin D status negatively affects muscular strength and power of collegiate athletes. Int J Sport Nutr Exerc Metab 2016;26(6):558–64.

79. McClung JP, Gaffney-Stomberg E, Lee JJ. Female athletes: a population at risk of vitamin and mineral deficiencies affecting health and performance. J Trace Elem Med Biol 2014;28(4):388–92.

80. Eskici G, Gunay M, Baltaci AK, et al. The effect of zinc supplementation on the urinary excretion of elements in female athletes. Pak J Pharm Sci 2016;29(1): 125–9.

81. Barrack MT, Van Loan MD, Rauh MJ, et al. Physiologic and behavioral indicators of energy deficiency in female adolescent runners with elevated bone turnover. Am J Clin Nutr 2010;92(3):652–9.

82. Lappe J, Cullen D, Haynatzki G, et al. Calcium and vitamin D supplementation decreases incidence of stress fractures in female navy recruits. J Bone Miner Res 2008;23(5):741–9.

83. Deldicque L, Francaux M. Recommendations for healthy nutrition in female endurance runners: an update. Front Nutr 2015;2:17.

84. Rodriguez NR, DiMarco NM, Langley S. Position of the American Dietetic Association, Dietitians of Canada, and the American College of Sports Medicine: nutrition and athletic performance. J Am Diet Assoc 2009;109(3):509–27.

85. Haakonssen EC, Ross ML, Knight EJ, et al. The effects of a calcium-rich pre-exercise meal on biomarkers of calcium homeostasis in competitive female cyclists: a randomised crossover trial. PLoS One 2015;10(5):e0123302.

86. Goolsby MA, Boniquit N. Bone health in athletes: the role of exercise, nutrition, and hormones. Sports Health 2017;9(2):108–17.

87. Nielsen FH, Lukaski HC. Update on the relationship between magnesium and exercise. Magnes Res 2006;19(3):180–9.

88. Petrović J, Stanić D, Dmitrašinović G, et al. Magnesium supplementation diminishes peripheral blood lymphocyte DNA oxidative damage in athletes and sedentary young men. Oxid Med Cell Longev 2016;2016:2019643.

89. Lukaski HC, Nielsen FH. Dietary magnesium depletion affects metabolic responses during submaximal exercise in postmenopausal women. J Nutr 2002; 132(5):930–5.

90. Volpe SL. Magnesium and the athlete. Curr Sports Med Rep 2015;14(4):279–83.

91. Monteiro CP, Matias CN, Bicho M, et al. Coordination between antioxidant defences might be partially modulated by magnesium status. Magnes Res 2017; 29(4):161–8.

92. Woolf K, LoBuono D, Manore M. B vitamins and the female athlete. In: Beals K, editor. Nutrition and the female athlete. 2013.

93. McClung JP, Gaffney-Stomberg E. Optimizing performance, health, and wellbeing: nutritional factors. Mil Med 2016;181(1 Suppl):86–91.

94. Gamage JP, De Silva AP, Nalliah AK, et al. Effects of dehydration on cricket specific skill performance in hot and humid conditions. Int J Sport Nutr Exerc Metab 2016;26(6):531–41.

95. Chapelle L, Tassignon B, Aerenhouts D, et al. The hydration status of elite youth female soccer players during an official tournament. J Sports Med Phys Fitness 2016. [Epub ahead of print].

96. Adams J, Kavouras S, Robillard J, et al. Fluid balance of adolescent swimmers during training. J Strength Cond Res 2016;30(3):621–5.

97. Magee PJ, Gallagher AM, McCormack JM. High prevalence of dehydration and inadequate nutritional knowledge among university and club level athletes. Int J Sport Nutr Exerc Metab 2017;27(2):158–68.

98. Wenner M, Stachenfeld N. Fluid and electrolyte requirements for female athletes. In: Beals K, editor. Nutrition for the female athlete. 2013.

99. Armstrong L, Johnson E, McKenzie A, et al. Endurance cyclist fluid intake, hydration status, thirst, and thermal sensations: gender differences. Int J Sport Nutr Exerc Metab 2016;26(2):161–7.

100. Sawka MN, Burke LM, Eichner ER, et al. American College of Sports Medicine position stand. Exercise and fluid replacement. Med Sci Sports Exerc 2007; 39(2):377–90.

101. Sommerfield LM, McAnulty SR, McBride JM, et al. Validity of urine specific gravity when compared with plasma osmolality as a measure of hydration status in male and female NCAA collegiate athletes. J Strength Cond Res 2016;30(8): 2219–25.

102. Matias CN, Júdice PB, Santos DA, et al. Suitability of bioelectrical based methods to assess water compartments in recreational and elite athletes. J Am Coll Nutr 2016;35(5):413–21.

103. van Wijck K, Lenaerts K, Grootjans J, et al. Physiology and pathophysiology of splanchnic hypoperfusion and intestinal injury during exercise: strategies for evaluation and prevention. Am J Physiol Gastrointest Liver Physiol 2012; 303(2):G155–68.

104. Maagaard L, Ankersen DV, Végh Z, et al. Follow-up of patients with functional bowel symptoms treated with a low FODMAP diet. World J Gastroenterol 2016;22(15):4009–19.

105. Miller KK. Mechanisms by which nutritional disorders cause reduced bone mass in adults. J Womens Health (Larchmt) 2003;12(2):145–50.

106. Black KE, Skidmore P, Brown RC. Case study: nutritional strategies of a cyclist with celiac disease during an ultraendurance race. Int J Sport Nutr Exerc Metab 2012;22(4):304–10.

107. Lis D, Stellingwerff T, Kitic CM, et al. No effects of a short-term gluten-free diet on performance in nonceliac athletes. Med Sci Sports Exerc 2015;47(12): 2563–70.

108. Herpertz-Dahlmann B, Seitz J, Baines J. Food matters: how the microbiome and gut-brain interaction might impact the development and course of anorexia nervosa. Eur Child Adolesc Psychiatry 2017. [Epub ahead of print].

109. Shriver L, Wollenberg G, Gates G. Prevalence of disordered eating and its association with emotion regulation in female college athletes. Int J Sport Nutr Exerc Metab 2016;26(3):240–8.

110. Pyne DB, West NP, Cox AJ, et al. Probiotics supplementation for athletes—clinical and physiological effects. Eur J Sport Sci 2015;15(1):63–72.

111. McArdle WD, Katch FI, Katch VL. Sports and exercise nutrition. 3rd edition. Philadelphia: Lippincott Williams & Wilkins; 2009.

112. Jeromson S, Gallagher IJ, Galloway SDR, et al. Omega-3 fatty acids and skeletal muscle health. Drugs 2015;13:6977–7004.

113. Hasadsri L, Wang BH, Lee JV, et al. Omega-3 fatty acids as a putative treatment for traumatic brain injury. J Neurotrauma 2013;30(11):897–906.

Gastrointestinal Conditions in the Female Athlete

Barry Kent Diduch, MD

KEYWORDS

- Athlete • Bariatric surgery • Celiac disease • Exercise • FODMAPs diet
- Inflammatory bowel disease • Intestinal microbiome • Irritable bowel syndrome

KEY POINTS

- Gastrointestinal (GI) symptoms are common in athletes. Moderate exercise can have benefits on these symptoms and diseases, whereas high-intensity training may negatively affect many of the GI problems commonly found in athletes.
- Irritable bowel syndrome (IBS) is the most common lower GI complaint in athletes with the diarrhea predominant variant the most common in women. A trial of a FODMAPs diet may be helpful for both the IBS and the gluten-sensitive athlete.
- Inflammatory bowel disease and celiac disease can affect the athlete's ability to absorb micronutrients and macronutrients. These diseases may impact performance related to their intestinal and extraintestinal symptoms.
- Bariatric surgery has become more common, with an increasing frequency of these individuals becoming highly active postsurgically. These patients face significant nutritional challenges to intense exercise and may benefit from the services of a sports-specific dietitian.

> More marathons are won or lost in the porta-toilets than at the dinner table.
> —Bill Rodgers, multiple NY and Boston Marathon winner[1]

INTRODUCTION

The frequency of gastrointestinal (GI) complaints in athletes is surprisingly common. Of athletes, 30% to 50% report GI symptoms during training,[1–3] yet the intensity of these symptoms and how much they affect exercise are not clear. Severe GI distress has been reported in 4% of marathoners and 32% of Ironman participants. Similarly, 7% of triathletes report having abandoned a race because of GI complaints.[1] Conditions that commonly plague the athlete can be classified as immune-mediated (celiac

Disclosure: Neither author nor his family members have any relevant financial relationships, directly or indirectly, referred to in this article.

Department of Sports Medicine, James Madison University, 261 Bluestone Drive MSC 2301, Harrisonburg, VA 24401, USA

E-mail address: diduchbk@jmu.edu

sportsmed.theclinics.com
0278-5919/17/© 2017 Elsevier Inc. All rights reserved.

disease), inflammatory (inflammatory bowel disease [IBD], which refers to either ulcerative colitis [UC] or Crohn disease [CD]), or functional (irritable bowel syndrome [IBS]). Although many of the GI problems encountered by athletes are not gender specific, IBS and celiac disease are more prevalent in women.[4,5] Women with either of the IBDs of UC or CD experience increased symptoms during their menstrual cycle, and the choice of contraception can further influence these hormonally related symptoms.[6,7] Understanding the effects of exercise on the mechanical structure of the GI system and the physiologic function helps the clinician with both diagnosis and management, including recommendations on participation in exercise and competition.

Anatomy and Physiology

From a structural perspective, the GI tract can be divided into 4 major areas: the upper GI area, which extends from the esophagus to the stomach; the hepatobiliary system; the small intestines; and the colon. Various sports impact these locations differently, depending on the sport-specific posture as well as the physiologic response to exercise, which alters the functions within each region.[1] For example, upper GI symptoms, such as nausea, vomiting, gastroesophageal reflux, and belching, are more common in cycling sports compared with running. This upper GI symptom predominance is attributed to the delayed gastric-emptying time in response to exercise as well as the mechanical effect of the forward-flexed biking posture.[1,3] Conversely, runners experience more lower GI symptoms of diarrhea, cramping, bleeding, and flatulence. These changes are related to a decreased vagal tone, increased adrenergic levels, prolonged profusion times, and mechanical jostling of the intestinal contents.[2]

Effects of Exercise

The effects of regular exercise are widespread, yet variable throughout the body. Regular exercise influences the vagal tone and balance of the sympathetic/parasympathetic nervous system.[8] Reliable exercise has been found to alter the vascular flow both during and after exercise.[1,9] Consistent physical activity has been associated with a decrease in the rates of IBD flares, gallbladder disease, and colon cancer.[9]

Regulation of the intestinal tract is achieved through a combination of neuroendocrine factors and their effect on blood flow. During exercise, the parasympathetic system downregulates while sympathetic tone increases, causing alpha receptor-driven vasoconstriction.[1,9] This vasoconstriction results in a reduction of splanchnic blood flow, in certain cases by up to 80% from baseline.[1] With the drop in parasympathetic activity, there is a reduction in esophageal peristalsis and lower esophageal sphincter tone, leading to an increase in reflux symptoms.[9] Regular moderate exercise attenuates this downregulation of the parasympathetic system[3] and can be detected indirectly by cardiac monitoring through observing variability in heart rate and within the electrocardiogram "R-R" interval. Moreover, this improved parasympathetic adaptation has been associated with enhanced gut-based neutrophil function and an anti-inflammatory effect.[9]

Not all the adaptations prove beneficial to the body though. The decreased vagal activity seen during exercise can continue into the postexercise recovery phase[8] and can slow the nutrient absorption function of the intestines. It can also delay the healing that is needed to the epithelium after exercise. Vagal tone can only recover after sufficient rest, such as tapering training intensity and volume. This downregulation of neuroendocrine, blood flow, and effective nutrient absorption may be a factor in overtraining symptoms.[8]

Intestinal Microbiome

The intestinal flora is extraordinarily diverse, and we are learning more about how this impacts the function of the whole body.[10] Moderate exercise increases this biodiversity and the prevalence of different species of bacteria. For example, regular exercise increases lactobacilli and butyrate-producing bacteria found in the large intestine. Butyrate is a preferred energy source for colonic epithelial cells.[11] Similarly, the *Akkermansia* species of bacteria, which exhibits properties of mucin degradation and thus improved barrier function and reduced inflammation, also multiplies with activity.[9,11] This change in barrier function has been shown in animal models to be associated with decreased rates of diabetes and obesity.[11] Dietary changes can also impact this biodiversity. Whey protein, for example, has been shown to enhance the microbiome composition.[9]

The human body adapts on a microscopic level to improve absorption of nutrients and to repair itself. The intestinal endothelium, aided by the tight junctions between its single layer of cells, serves as a gateway for nutrient absorption and as a first-level barrier to toxins and pathogens.[12] The integrity of these cellular junctions may be impaired by many of the stresses resulting from intense exercise, such as dehydration and thermal injury.[8] In addition, prolonged or intense exercise decreases vagal tone, which is hypothesized to lead to decreased tight junction function, thus allowing for increased permeability of endotoxins and pathogens.[9] In a recent study, 81% of ultramarathoners were found to have increased levels of circulating endotoxins.[11] Although there still exists gaps in the understanding of this intricate system, there appears to be a synergy between diet, exercise, and metabolism, with the microbiome being a linchpin in this process.

Food-Dependent Anaphylaxis

The integrity of the gut epithelium comes into play with food-dependent anaphylaxis. There exists a subset of this condition observed in exercise: food-dependent exercise-induced anaphylaxis (FDEIA).[13] The pathophysiology of this phenomenon occurs across multiple organ systems, beginning in the gut. In response to exercise, there is a decrease in gastric acid production and therefore a decline in the breakdown and digestion of antigens.[14] Meanwhile, the epithelial tight junctions become "leaky" in response to exercise, resulting in increased antigen absorption. Furthermore, the enhanced perfusion to the skin during exercise delivers a higher concentration of these antigens to the epidermis, where phenotypically unique mast cells reside. All these factors combined allow allergen levels to reach a crucial threshold, triggering an allergic response[13] clinically expressed as exercise-induced bronchospasm, urticaria, or even anaphylaxis. Foods associated with this FDEIA spectrum include the common allergens: cereals, seafood, peanut, tree nuts, egg, milk, and even vegetables.[13,14]

Upper Gastrointestinal Symptoms

Esophageal reflux is the number one upper GI complaint in athletes.[3] Up to 50% of athletes will have upper GI symptoms during training, with certain sports having a higher prevalence than others.[3] Acid reflux, vomiting, and gastritis are thought to be related to mechanical, neurologic, and vascular contributors. Weightlifters complain of reflux or vomiting more often than runners or cyclists,[15] which is thought to be due to the abdominal straining required for the sport.[3,16] On the other hand, reflux symptoms experienced by cyclists are attributed to body positioning.[3,16] Neurologically, one must once again consider that the sympathetic response takes precedence during exercise. Consequently, parasympathetic tone decreases during, as well as following, bouts of exercise, leading to delayed gastric emptying and an increase in gastric contents available for reflux.[17] Vascular causes are the third major component. Endurance athletes exhibit a significantly reduced splanchnic flow theorized to lead to higher rates of gastric mucosal breakdown. Indeed, Choi and colleagues[18] found 22 of 24 professional long-distance runners had at least one mucosal lesion on endoscopy.

Treatment of upper GI conditions for athletes should focus on lifestyle changes before considering medication management. Avoiding solid food and high carbohydrate drinks before exercise sessions may prove helpful.[16] In addition, limiting the carbohydrate concentration of sports drinks to 6% to 8% during training will allow the athlete to optimize carbohydrate absorption and assist with gastric emptying, while minimizing GI distress.[19] Refraining from the common practice of preparticipation nonsteroidal inflammatory drug (NSAID) use is also protective. NSAIDs, via their mechanism of action, reduce splanchnic blood flow and disrupt mucosal integrity.[1] Safe medication options such as H2 blockers or proton-pump inhibitors (PPIs) may be used if needed before exercise or for short treatment intervals when GI symptoms arise.

Gallbladder Disease

The sympathetic/parasympathetic adaptation that occurs with regular exercise may have a similar effect on biliary function, but there is a significant lack of research in this area. A limited study of marathoners demonstrated elevated cholecystokinin levels before and after a race, suggesting increased gallbladder emptying.[20] Conversely, in another study, recumbent cycling at 65% maximum effort demonstrated no effect on gallbladder motility.[21] Studies of regular exercisers have shown mixed or statistically insignificant changes in gallbladder function and no changes to gallstone formation.[20,22] A review by Shephard, however, showed that there was indeed a reduction in both gallbladder disease and gallbladder cancer with regular exercise.[20]

Ischemic Colitis

Splanchnic blood flow can be significantly affected by exercise and is regulated both intrinsically and extrinsically. Within the splanchnic system, the response to exercise includes a myogenic increase in tone due to upregulation in adrenergic smooth muscle activity leading to a decrease in blood flow.[8] Locally produced vasoactive substances, such as gastrin, secretin, and cholecystokinin, lead to even less perfusion due to vasoconstriction.[23] At rest, the liver receives an estimated 25% to 30% of the circulating blood flow, but during moderate-intensity exercise (Vo_2 max of 70%), this splanchnic flow has been found to decrease by up to 80%.[24] This degree of shunting toward skeletal muscle and skin may be even higher in untrained individuals, warmer exercise environments, and increasing levels of dehydration.[1] This redistribution leaves a state of relative hypoperfusion of the intestines, which, if prolonged, can lead to ischemia of varying extent.[1,24] Mild effects include decreased nutrient absorption during exercise, delayed gastric emptying, cramping, or nausea,[24] whereas more severe manifestations include mucosal erosions, gastritis, and ischemic colitis.[25]

This decreased blood flow can additionally affect the actual absorption rate of oral rehydration efforts. When exercising at 85% Vo_2 max, cyclists have been found to have their fluid absorption limited to 0.5 L per hour.[26] This limited rehydration rate during exercise results in any extra volume intake to remain in the stomach and small intestines, manifested as athlete bloating. More severe effects include mucosal integrity breakdown, epithelial damage, and tight junction degradation, all of which may lead to occult or overt blood loss. Baska and colleagues[27] found 85% of ultramarathoners tested positive for occult blood after a 161-km event. The risk of splanchnic ischemia is greater in the dehydrated athlete (>4% body weight loss), female athlete, younger-aged athlete, higher-intensity activities, and vertical impact sports.[24] There exist reports of pancolitis and infarctions that required colectomy following a marathon.[25] Less strongly associated with this ischemia are dietary factors and previous abdominal surgery. NSAIDs, too, can further reduce splanchnic blood flood and cause increased endothelial damage during exercise, but the extent of this effect is not clearly understood.[1,28]

Bariatric Surgery Athlete

Coincident with the obesity epidemic, the rate of bariatric surgery has steadily increased over the years, surpassing the 200,000 annual procedure mark in 2007.[29] For those who undergo gastric bypass surgery, 6% will become highly physically active after surgery[30]; thus, this population poses a significant challenge for the sports medicine clinician. Providing advice on exercise and nutrition can be complicated in a healthy athlete, but this becomes exponentially more difficult and complex within this cohort.

One such reason contributing to the challenge is the actual term "bariatric surgery." The term "bariatric surgery" encompasses a wide variety of interventions ranging from banding or intragastric ballooning (restrictive procedures) to the more complex sleeves and rerouting procedures such as a Roux-en-Y. Each carries its own associated effects on the digestive system often in the form of early satiety, restriction, and malabsorption.[29] The physician must be aware of the details of the actual completed procedures, paying particular attention to the nuances of the postsurgical anatomy because this will certainly offer clues regarding the potential functional and nutritional complications.

Many of the recommendations bariatric patients receive following surgery do not coincide well with the exercise recommended for attaining weight loss or maintenance.[31] For example, these patients are often recommended to limit premeal and postmeal fluid intake to avoid overfilling. Overfilling results in nausea, vomiting, and dumping syndrome due to volume intolerance.[29] Nevertheless, the exercising individual has needs that contradict these routine measures, and ingesting an appropriate amount of fluid may be difficult. It is recommended that the patient attempt 12 oz of fluid intake per hour during the day to maintain adequate hydration; however, this amount would be inadequate during intense, prolonged activity or exercise in a hot environment.[30,31]

This same, now-limited gastric volume limits the ingestion of macronutrients, specifically protein and carbohydrates.[31,32] Moreover, postsurgical patients are instructed to consume protein before carbohydrates, which, in turn, limits their energy availability for exercise[32] (**Box 1**). In order to continue postsurgical weight loss, the exercising bariatric patient may require twice the normal protein intake needs normally recommended. This protein/carbohydrate balance is difficult to do successfully, because carbohydrates play a vital role for fueling exercise as well as to replenish glycogen stores. Finding a delicate balance between consuming enough high levels of protein, fueling the body with the needed carbohydrates, and not overfilling the gastric volume is a constant struggle with this population.

On a smaller scale, the absorption of micronutrients is influenced by postsurgical anatomic changes. Postprocedure patients are often recommended a daily PPI given the increased risk of developing gastroduodenal ulcers.[32] This class of medication can

> **Box 1**
> **Bariatric surgery and the athlete**
>
> Some procedures are restrictive based, whereas others are malabsorptive. This will influence recommendations for micronutrient and macronutrient intake.
>
> Adequate hydration can be difficult. Recommend 12 oz of fluid intake per hour throughout the day with extra intake for intense, prolonged, or hot training days.
>
> Protein intake needs may be twice as high as normal recommendations. Work closely with a sports-specific dietitian to meet nutrition goals for training level.
>
> Monitor and replace micronutrients: vitamin B12, folate, vitamin D, and ferritin.

impair vitamin B12 absorption, as well as impact the intestinal microbiome discussed above. PPIs historically have also been associated with hypomagnesemia, although recent findings refute this claim. Other common nutrient deficiencies following surgery include water-soluble vitamins (folate, thiamine), vitamin D, and iron.[29]

During a patient encounter, the sports medicine clinician must take into consideration all of the volume, hydration, and absorption complications common to these patients. As such, the physician may recommend a sweat rate calculation to better develop a unique hydration plan geared toward the specific patient and the surgical procedure completed.[29] A sweat rate calculation involves having the patient weigh himself in minimal clothing before and after an hour of strenuous exercise to determine their unique sweat rate. These data help the clinician individualize the necessary hydration goals leading up to and following exercise. In addition, while considering the absorption changes, the physician should consider obtaining laboratory assessment of micronutrient levels to more objectively derive supplementation and dietary recommendations. Last, it may be helpful to consult the services of a sport-specific dietitian for added expertise beyond that of the assigned postoperative bariatric care team.

Celiac Disease/Nonceliac Gluten Sensitivity

Gluten is a protein found in grains, particularly wheat, rye, and barley. Sensitivity to this protein can cause several different types of immune reactions.[33,34] Celiac disease is an autoimmune condition in which the body reacts to ingested gluten in the small intestine. Damage occurs to the villi leading to increased epithelial permeability and decreased micronutrient absorption.[33] Celiac disease is diagnosed by clinical symptoms combined with either positive antibodies (tissue transglutaminase and antiendomysial antibodies) or biopsy of the small intestine. This condition affects 1% to 1.5% of the US population, with women having a 2.5 greater incidence than men.[33] Approximately 0.1% of the US population has a diagnosed wheat allergy, yet it is reported that 5% to 10% of individuals exhibit a gluten sensitivity without antibody presence.[33,35] This antibody negative state is referred to as *Nonceliac Gluten Sensitivity* (NCGS), and affected individuals will respond positively to a gluten-free diet. The common symptoms of these gluten sensitivity syndromes include chronic diarrhea, abdominal bloating/cramping, fatigue, and micronutrient deficiencies.[33] Specifically, the B vitamins, iron, vitamin D, and calcium are not absorbed appropriately, potentially leading to conditions such as vitamin B12 deficiency, iron deficiency, and osteopenia/osteoporosis. The affected, blunted villi also exhibit an accompanying decline in macronutrient absorption, which can lead to an energy deficit and prolonged recovery in the training athlete.[35] Altered absorption conditions change the microflora of the intestinal tract, disrupting the epithelium.[35] Similar damage can occur from the simultaneous decrease in splanchnic perfusion from high-intensity exercise.[8,34] The ensuing integrity loss of the epithelium allows for the gluten proteins to be absorbed to higher amounts, leading to increased sensitivity in the NCGS population.[13,14]

When managing an athlete with celiac disease, the provider should assess the micronutrient and macronutrient status. Regular monitoring of vitamin B12, ferritin, and vitamin D is essential.[33] Meeting the protein and carbohydrate goals needed for high-intensity training can be difficult on a gluten-free diet.[36] The skill set of a registered dietitian may be beneficial to help optimize energy availability for activity as well as recovery. Furthermore, educating the athlete's family, coaching staff, and support staff is important to prevent the cross-contamination of meals and team snacks. Other challenges arise for the athlete, such as locating gluten-free alternatives during team travel. Overall, individuals tend to respond well to gluten-free diets because the offending agent has been removed and clinical improvement should follow.[35] Tracking antibody levels is an additional option to confirm disease response to a gluten-free diet.[33]

Although the estimated population of individuals affected by gluten is 5% to 10%, there has been an explosion in athletes following gluten-free diets at their own choosing.[35,37] Lis and colleagues[37] conducted a survey of 910 athletes, including recreational, Olympic, and professional individuals, and comprising 58% women. Forty-one percent of this population had chosen to eat a gluten-free diet at least 50% of the time. Of these individuals, 70% were endurance athletes. Lis went on to note that most of the gluten-free athletes, 57%, were self-diagnosed as "gluten sensitive," whereas only 10% were formally diagnosed as NCGS. Interestingly, this value correlates with the general population. Of those that had opted for a gluten-free diet, 81% reported improved GI symptoms of less bloating, gas, diarrhea, and decreased fatigue and believed performance improved as well. In a follow-up study, nonceliac, non-gluten-sensitive athletes were enrolled in a double-blind placebo-controlled crossover study in which a gluten-free diet was provided to all participants.[38] One subset was the given an additional gluten-containing protein bar, whereas the other group received a gluten-free bar for 7 days. The athletes' performance on a 15-minute bicycle time trial was subsequently measured. The investigators found no statistical difference between the 2 treatment arms.[38]

Non-celiac-, non-gluten-sensitive athletes who choose to follow a gluten-free diet raise several concerns for the clinician. The common belief that this nutritional plan will lead to improved performance lacks evidence.[37–39] The restricted diet carries a risk of micronutrient and macronutrient deficiency with the possibility of orthorexia nervosa practices in pursuit of a healthy diet.[37] There may also exist a subset of these individuals who experience true relief either because of subclinical gluten sensitivity exacerbated by high levels of exercise or by associated dietary antigens.[13,14,35] Furthermore, it is possible the athletes that self-select a gluten-free diet suffer from poorly absorbed food antigens and would respond to a diet low in fermentable oligosaccharides, disaccharides, monosaccharides, and polyols (FODMAPs diet).[40] Helping athletes appropriately implement a FODMAPs diet can be challenging and requires the assistance of a sports dietitian (**Table 1**).

Inflammatory Bowel Disease

IBD affects approximately 1 in 500 Americans with an equal distribution between men and women.[6] The title of "IBD" encompasses the 2 different pathologic conditions of UC and CD; both autoimmune mediated. UC is a shallow mucosal inflammatory disease of the colon that propagates in a continuous fashion proximally from the anus. CD is a deeper, transmural inflammatory process with discontinuous patches of disease throughout the GI tract anywhere from the mouth to the anus. The diagnosis

Table 1
Fermentable oligosaccharides, disaccharides, monosaccharides, and polyols diet: foods to avoid

Oligosaccharides	Disaccharides	Monosaccharides	Polyols
Grains (wheat, rye, barley); garlic; onions; beans and other legumes	Milk; yogurt; ice cream; soft cheeses	Apples; artichokes; asparagus; mango; peaches; pears, peas; high-fructose corn syrup; honey	Apples; apricots; blackberries; cauliflower; mushrooms; plums; prunes; mannitol, polydextrose, sorbitol, xylitol

Phase 1: Elimination of as many FODMAPs foods as possible for 7 days.
Phase 2: Reintroduction or challenge phase. Introduce a different group at 3-day intervals.
Phase 3: Maintenance phase. Limit triggering foods identified in phase 2 while meeting micronutrient and macronutrient needs.
Data from Lis D, Ahuja KD, Stellingwerff T, et al. Food avoidance in athletes: FODMAP foods on the list. Appl Physiol Nutr Metab 2016;41(9):1002–4; and Lis D, Ahuja KD, Stellingwerff T, et al. Case study: utilizing a low FODMAP diet to combat exercise-induced gastrointestinal symptoms. Int J Sport Nutr Exerc Metab 2016;26(5):481–7.

of IBD is confirmed by antibody testing and colonoscopic biopsies.[6] Common symptoms include arthralgias (40%–50%)[41] and arthritis (15%–20% in CD; and 10% in UC).[6] The arthritis tends to present in 2 different patterns: as a large joint oligoarthritis involving the knees, ankles, wrists, elbows, and hips or as spinal ankylosing spondylitis.[6] Although the arthritis is inflammatory, it is not erosive or deforming. Those individuals who develop arthritis are more likely to have the HLA-B27 or HLA-DR103 phenotypes on genetic testing.[42]

There are limited studies looking at the role of exercise in IBD.[43] DeFilippis and colleagues[41] surveyed 227 patients with IBD, 65% of whom were women, to assess exercise levels while living with this disease. Twenty-four percent of the respondents exercised 2 to 4 times weekly, whereas 18% exercised more than 4 times a week. Of these regular exercisers, 51% reported moderate levels of exercise and 16% were vigorous exercisers. Most of the responders were in a controlled state of their disease. Despite this, 44% reported that their exercise was limited by their disease because of fatigue, joint pain, GI symptoms, or embarrassment.[43] Bilski and colleagues[44] performed a systematic literature review investigating what effect, if any, exercise had on the quality of life of patients with IBD as well as disease activity. Moderate exercise was found to be well tolerated and led to improved quality-of-life measurements as well as reduced stress levels. However, there were no favorable effects observed specifically regarding the disease activity.[44] Bilski went on to postulate that the generalized positive effects observed with this exercise was likely attributed to the release of anti-inflammatory myokines from muscle, whereas the decrease in visceral fat was due to local proinflammatory effects on the intestinal epithelium.[43,44] Last, Ploeger and colleagues[45] compared a group of 15 pediatric patients specifically with CD. On 2 separate occasions, blood was analyzed for inflammatory cells, cytokines, and growth factors (ie, tumor necrosis factor-alpha, insulin-like growth factor-1) at points before, during, and after moderate- or high-intensity exercise. No observable differences were noted between the 2 exercise sessions on any of the measured markers.

As discussed above, high-intensity or endurance exercise potentially leads to significant decreases in splanchnic blood flow, which in turn increases damage to the intestinal epithelium, increasing the absorption of antigenic bacteria through a leaky gut.[8,45] To date, there are no data investigating the role of high-intensity exercise in inducing clinical IBD, disease-related arthritis, or worsening IBD disease state.

The clinician caring for the athlete with IBD should be prepared to manage the GI and musculoskeletal symptoms.[6] Intestinal inflammation leads to malabsorption of micronutrients and macronutrients. Vitamin B12 and iron deficiencies are common and affect performance. Assessing for vitamin D deficiency, osteopenia, and overall risk of stress fractures should be completed to intervene expeditiously.[6] Certain common IBD symptoms, such as bloating, diarrhea, and cramping, may require medication or dietary modifications to allow for physical activity and sports participation.

IBD can affect female athletes in specific ways that differ from their male counterparts. Because of the effects of required abdominal surgeries for IBD, resultant fistulae, and/or fecal incontinence, there is a higher percentage of women with a negative body image compared with men.[46] Similarly, women with IBD report a lower rate of sexual activity secondary to abdominal pain and fear of fecal incontinence.[46] Fertility rates in IBD patients are reduced, but this appears to be voluntary.[46] The treating clinician may recommend pregnancy, careful family planning, or even avoidance given concerns regarding the medicines used to manage the IBD. The medicines used in IBD are variable in their safety profiles. For example, biologic agents are not contraindicated during pregnancy, whereas methotrexate should be avoided because of its teratogenic risk.[46] Contraceptive choices are based on patient preference and risk of thromboembolic events. For those women with moderate or severe IBD disease, progesterone-only preparations may be preferred to combined estrogen/progesterone contraceptives.[46]

IRRITABLE BOWEL SYNDROME

IBS affects 10% to 15% of the population and is twice as likely to affect women as men.[4,44] IBS is thought to be a functional problem of altered GI motility, abnormal secretory function, and visceral hypersensitivity mediated by both the central and enteric nervous systems.[47] It is associated with psychological conditions such as anxiety or depression and is more prevalent in those with a history of prior sexual or physical abuse.[48] There is some evidence that an unfavorable gut microbiome may play a role in the development of IBS.[49] Common symptoms of IBS include abdominal distention, abdominal pain, a change in stool pattern, passage of clear mucus, and symptoms worsen before, or are relieved by, defecation.[44] Other extraintestinal manifestations include dyspepsia, headaches, fibromyalgia, pelvic pain, palpitations, sleep disturbances, and chronic fatigue syndrome.[49] Besides these frequent symptoms, women with IBS report more severe flares throughout different phases of their menstrual cycle. These cyclical flares are thought to be due to sex hormone receptors along the GI tract that may mediate the visceral pain and GI transit time. In a retrospective study of more than 90,000 women, Bird and colleagues[50] found the risk of developing IBS was elevated in women taking drospirenone-containing oral contraceptives compared with levonorgestrel (hazard ratio 1.7; number needed to harm 4). Furthermore, a meta-analysis by Adeyemo and colleagues[5] found that women more often reported visceral pain, flatulence, and disturbance in stool patterns during premenstruation and menstruation as compared with midcycle symptoms.

There exist 3 subtypes of IBS: constipation-predominant (IBS-C), diarrhea-predominant (IBS-D), and mixed type. All are associated with symptoms related to defecation (**Table 2**). The diagnosis of IBS is based on both the presence of features and the absence of "red flag" symptoms. The Rome Criteria aids in the clinical diagnosis.[51] Rome IV requires symptoms be present a minimum of 6 months, with weekly symptoms consistently occurring over the prior 3 months. For IBS-C, a decrease in the frequency of bowel movements to less than 3 times a week must be present.

Table 2
Irritable bowel syndrome evaluation

I: Inquire	B: Background	S: Sinister Features
• Abdominal pain/discomfort at least 1 d a week for the past 3 mo • Symptoms worsened before or relieved after a bowel movement • Symptoms associated with a change in stool character: firm, large, lumpy OR loose, watery, mucus • Symptoms associated with a change in stool frequency	• Family history of IBS, IBD, celiac disease, or cancer • Food sensitivity • Adequate fiber intake in diet • History of physical or sexual abuse	• Unintentional weight loss • Severe diarrhea or constipation • Occult or gross blood in stool • Onset after 50 y old • Recent travel or outdoor activity associated with possible intestinal parasitic infection • Nocturnal symptoms • Abnormal abdominal examination

Data from Chey WD, Kurlander J, Eswaran S. Irritable bowel syndrome: a clinical review. JAMA 2015;313(9):949–58.

Alternatively, for IBS-D to be considered, stooling frequency must surpass 3 movements a day. Worrisome "red flag" findings include the onset of symptoms after age 50, unexplained weight loss, nocturnal diarrhea, rectal bleeding, and unexplained iron deficiency, and require further investigation into alternative causes including malignancy.

The differential of IBS is extensive and includes IBD, celiac disease, diverticulitis, parasitic infection, tumor, thyroid disorder, and others.[49] History, physical examination, and basic laboratory work can be used to identify potential sinister signs, or "red flags," indicating an increased probability of an alternate diagnosis.[51] Basic laboratory studies should include a complete blood count, erythrocyte sedimentation rate, chemistry panel, thyroid stimulating hormone, and fecal occult blood test.[4,49] Menees and colleagues[52] performed a meta-analysis to see if C-reactive protein, erythrocyte sedimentation rate, fecal calprotectin, or fecal lactoferrin could be used to differentiate between IBS, IBD, and normal subjects. They found that a C-reactive protein level less than 0.5 or fecal calprotectin less than 40 was correlated with the diagnosis of IBS. In their analysis, erythrocyte sedimentation rate and fecal lactoferrin were not statistically useful. This study did not look at regularly exercising individuals and how exercise may influence these laboratory values. For IBS-D, celiac disease should be strongly considered in the differential, and testing for tissue transglutaminase antibodies is warranted.[49] In the absence of any red flags and with the Rome Criteria being met, there is a positive predictive value of 98%, or less than a 1% chance of an alternate diagnosis.[4]

The usefulness of the Rome Criteria and laboratory studies has not been studied in the athletic population. Other factors associated with exercise can modify stool patterns. The prevalence of occult GI blood loss due to exercise can be significant.[27] In addition, the gut microbiome can be altered by intense exercise, resulting in changes in stool patterns. These features complicate the evaluation and management of IBS in the athletic population.[53]

Exercise is sometimes the recommended treatment of IBS 50 because it can improve GI transit time and bloating symptoms in IBS-C patients.[54] On the other hand, exercise can produce unfavorable effects in IBS-D individuals.[4,47] Johannesson and colleagues[55] performed a randomized controlled trial involving 75 patients with

IBS (no differentiation between IBS subtypes) and monitored the response to regular, moderate exercise. One group exercised 20 to 60 minutes, 3 to 5 days a week, whereas the control group continued their regular activities. After 12 weeks, 43% of the exercise group claimed improved symptoms, whereas only 8% complained of a worsening. Within the control group, only 26% had improvement, whereas 23% reported worsened symptoms. As such, it is thought regular, moderate exercise may be beneficial in IBS. High-intensity or prolonged exercise still needs further evaluation to determine its impact on IBS.

Management of IBS can be divided into treating the symptoms and regulating the bowel pattern.[49] Bloating, spasms, and pain can be managed with antispasmodic agents, such as hyoscyamine or dicyclomine.[47] These medicines may have anticholinergic side effects that are particularly concerning to athletes, including dry mouth, dizziness, somnolence, or heat intolerance. Peppermint oil capsules relax intestinal smooth muscle and decrease pain and bloating, with the most common adverse event being heartburn.[47] Antidepressants may play a role in both intestinal and systemic symptoms of IBS. Tricyclic antidepressants have shown better efficacy than selective serotonin reuptake inhibitors, especially in IBS-D patients.[47,49]

Some IBS patients, especially those with diarrhea predominance, may obtain relief with a gluten-free diet.[40,49] This relief-by-avoidance notion has been expanded to include other poorly absorbed agents in the FODMAPs diet: fermentable oligosaccharides, disaccharides, and polyols.[39] The FODMAPs diet goes beyond the low-gluten diet and has been shown to be efficacious in both IBS-C and IBS-D patients.[49] The athletic population may find it difficult to meet micronutrient and macronutrient needs by following a FODMAPs diet long term and may need the assistance of a sports dietitian. Although a FODMAPs diet is thought to improve the contributory malabsorption problems, it may also negatively affect the gut microbiome. To date, there are very limited studies looking at the effects of a FODMAPs diet in athletes, although this diet is becoming more popular in endurance athletes, much as a gluten-free diet.[35]

Regulating the stool pattern of IBS may be helpful in managing both the symptoms and the syndrome's impact on an athlete's activities.[49] Constipation-predominant patients can be provided osmotic laxatives, such as polyethylene glycol, or a guanylate cyclase-c agonist, such as linaclotide. These medicines can be titrated to achieve the desired bowel frequency. For IBS-D patients, the tricyclic antidepressants loperamide and alosteron have been shown to decrease the frequency of stools, although some of the side effects are serious (**Table 3**).[47]

Table 3
Management of irritable bowel syndrome in the athlete

Management Questions	Diet	Spasm/Pain	Constipation	Diarrhea
• How does the IBS affect the athlete? • How does the training affect the IBS? • What effect does menstruation have on the IBS?	• Maintain adequate fiber and fluid intake • Consider: ○ Gluten-free diet ○ FODMAPs diet	• Hyoscyamine • Dicyclomine • Peppermint oil • Tricyclic antidepressants	• Polyethylene glycol • Linaclotide	• Loperamide • Alosetron

> **Box 2**
> **General recommendations**
>
> During regular training, maintain normal amounts of dietary fiber but reduce fiber intake on competition day
>
> Limit carbohydrate concentration of hydration fluid to less than 10% and consider a mixed glucose/fructose fluid if symptoms persist
>
> Hydration rates may be limited to 0.5 L/h during intense exercise, so hydrate well beforehand
>
> NSAIDs may have a negative effect on the gastrointestinal system during exercise and should be avoided beforehand if possible

SUMMARY

Both upper and lower GI problems occur in athletes with 25% to 50% of recreational athletes and up to 70% of elite athletes reporting either upper or lower GI symptoms affecting training/competition.[2,3] Gastroesophageal reflux and IBS are the 2 most common diagnoses. Although celiac disease and IBS occur more frequently in women, many of the GI conditions that occur in athletes are not sex specific.[48] In women, menstrual cycle hormonal changes have been noted to affect the symptoms of both IBS and IBD.[7]

The clinician should consider several factors when evaluating an athlete with GI complaints. These factors include the mechanical forces specific to the training, altered splanchnic blood flow during and after training, and neuroendocrine changes that can linger long after training.[1] The intestinal microbiome, too, plays a crucial role in intestinal well-being and is affected by regular, intense exercise. As such, the clinician should consider evaluation of micronutrient and macronutrient levels.[9] It is important to inquire about exercise and eating practices because this may reveal contributors to the GI distress. Some frequent offenders include certain food types and timing related to exercise, exercise intensity, and medication use (**Box 2**).

Management of GI complaints depends on whether the upper or lower sections are involved and often do not require medications. For example, to alleviate reflux, the clinician should recommend modifying the preexercise food volume and carbohydrate concentration.[3] On the other hand, IBD symptoms can be modified simply by changing the intensity of the exercise. A trial of a FODMAPs diet may be a good first step in managing IBS patients or suspected cases of gluten sensitivity.[40] As with any dietary adaptations, extra attention should be given to make sure adequate carbohydrate, protein, and micronutrients are maintained to meet the needs of exercising individuals. Regardless of the symptoms, having a good working understanding of the human GI system will help the clinician provide better care and advice, particularly to the athlete population, because exercise is an influencing factor. By doing so, the athlete and physician align toward the same goal: to keep the athlete exercising safely.

REFERENCES

1. de Oliveira EP, Burini RC, Jeukendrup A. Gastrointestinal complaints during exercise: prevalence, etiology, and nutritional recommendations. Sports Med 2014; 44(Suppl 1):S79–85.
2. Ho GW. Lower gastrointestinal distress in endurance athletes. Curr Sports Med Rep 2009;8(2):85–91.

3. Waterman JJ, Kapur R. Upper gastrointestinal issues in athletes. Curr Sports Med Rep 2012;11(2):99–104.
4. Heiman DL, Lishnak TS, Trojian TH. Irritable bowel syndrome in athletes and exercise. Curr Sports Med Rep 2008;7(2):100–3.
5. Adeyemo MA, Spiegel BM, Chang L. Meta-analysis: do irritable bowel syndrome symptoms vary between men and women? Aliment Pharmacol Ther 2010;32(6):738–55.
6. Zakaria AA, Rifat SF. Inflammatory bowel disease: concerns for the athlete. Curr Sports Med Rep 2008;7(2):104–7.
7. Bharadwaj S, Barber MD, Graff LA, et al. Symptomatology of irritable bowel syndrome and inflammatory bowel disease during the menstrual cycle. Gastroenterol Rep (Oxf) 2015;3(3):185–93.
8. Van Houten JM, Wessells RJ, Lujan HL, et al. My gut feeling says rest: increased intestinal permeability contributes to chronic diseases in high-intensity exercisers. Med Hypotheses 2015;85(6):882–6.
9. Cronin O, Molloy MG, Shanahan F. Exercise, fitness, and the gut. Curr Opin Gastroenterol 2016;32(2):67–73.
10. Cresci GA, Bawden E. Gut microbiome: what we do and don't know. Nutr Clin Pract 2015;30(6):734–46.
11. Cook MD, Allen JM, Pence BD, et al. Exercise and gut immune function: evidence of alterations in colon immune cell homeostasis and microbiome characteristics with exercise training. Immunol Cell Biol 2016;94(2):158–63.
12. Lamprecht M, Frauwallner A. Exercise, intestinal barrier dysfunction and probiotic supplementation. Med Sport Sci 2012;59:47–56.
13. Morita E, Chinuki Y, Takahashi H. Recent advances of in vitro tests for the diagnosis of food-dependent exercise-induced anaphylaxis. J Dermatol Sci 2013;71(3):155–9.
14. Wong GK, Krishna MT. Food-dependent exercise-induced anaphylaxis: is wheat unique? Curr Allergy Asthma Rep 2013;13(6):639–44.
15. Collings KL, Pierce Pratt F, Rodriguez-Stanley S, et al. Esophageal reflux in conditioned runners, cyclists, and weightlifters. Med Sci Sports Exerc 2003;35(5):730–5.
16. Simons SM, Kennedy RG. Gastrointestinal problems in runners. Curr Sports Med Rep 2004;3(2):112–6.
17. Brouns F, Beckers E. Is the gut an athletic organ? Digestion, absorption and exercise. Sports Med 1993;15(4):242–57.
18. Choi SC, Choi SJ, Kim JA, et al. The role of gastrointestinal endoscopy in long-distance runners with gastrointestinal symptoms. Eur J Gastroenterol Hepatol 2001;13(9):1089–94.
19. Parmelee-Peters K, Moeller JL. Gastroesophageal reflux in athletes. Curr Sports Med Rep 2004;3(2):107–11.
20. Shephard RJ. Physical activity and the biliary tract in health and disease. Sports Med 2015;45(9):1295–309.
21. Utter AC, Goss FL, Whitcomb DC, et al. The effects of acute exercise on gallbladder function in an adult female population. Med Sci Sports Exerc 1996;28(3):280–4.
22. Friedman GD, Kannel WB, Dawber TR. The epidemiology of gallbladder disease: observations in the Framingham study. J Chronic Dis 1966;19(3):273–92.
23. Granger DN, Holm L, Kvietys P. The gastrointestinal circulation: physiology and pathophysiology. Compr Physiol 2015;5(3):1541–83.

24. de Oliveira EP, Burini RC. Food-dependent, exercise-induced gastrointestinal distress. J Int Soc Sports Nutr 2011;8:12.
25. Eichner ER. Ischemic colitis in athletes. Curr Sports Med Rep 2011;10(5):242–3.
26. Jeukendrup AE, Jentjens RL, Moseley L. Nutritional considerations in triathlon. Sports Med 2005;35(2):163–81.
27. Baska RS, Moses FM, Graeber G, et al. Gastrointestinal bleeding during an ultra-marathon. Dig Dis Sci 1990;35(2):276–9.
28. Van Wijck K, Lenaerts K, Van Bijnen AA, et al. Aggravation of exercise-induced intestinal injury by ibuprofen in athletes. Med Sci Sports Exerc 2012;44(12): 2257–62.
29. Petering R, Webb CW. Exercise, fluid, and nutrition recommendations for the postgastric bypass exerciser. Curr Sports Med Rep 2009;8(2):92–7.
30. Clark N. Case study: nutrition challenges of a marathon runner with a gastric bypass. Int J Sport Nutr Exerc Metab 2011;21(6):515–9.
31. Marchesi F, De Sario G, Reggiani V, et al. Road running after gastric bypass for morbid obesity: rationale and results of a new protocol. Obes Surg 2015;25(7): 1162–70.
32. McMahon MM, Sarr MG, Clark MM, et al. Clinical management after bariatric surgery: value of a multidisciplinary approach. Mayo Clin Proc 2006;81(10 Suppl): S34–45.
33. Mancini LA, Trojian T, Mancini AC. Celiac disease and the athlete. Curr Sports Med Rep 2011;10(2):105–8.
34. Scherf KA, Brockow K, Biedermann T, et al. Wheat-dependent exercise-induced anaphylaxis. Clin Exp Allergy 2016;46(1):10–20.
35. Lis DM, Fell JW, Ahuja KD, et al. Commercial hype versus reality: our current scientific understanding of gluten and athletic performance. Curr Sports Med Rep 2016;15(4):262–8.
36. Black KE, Skidmore P, Brown RC. Case study: nutritional strategies of a cyclist with celiac disease during an ultraendurance race. Int J Sport Nutr Exerc Metab 2012;22(4):304–10.
37. Lis DM, Stellingwerff T, Shing CM, et al. Exploring the popularity, experiences, and beliefs surrounding gluten-free diets in nonceliac athletes. Int J Sport Nutr Exerc Metab 2015;25(1):37–45.
38. Lis D, Stellingwerff T, Kitic CM, et al. No effects of a short-term gluten-free diet on performance in nonceliac athletes. Med Sci Sports Exerc 2015;47(12):2563–70.
39. Lis D, Ahuja KD, Stellingwerff T, et al. Food avoidance in athletes: FODMAP foods on the list. Appl Physiol Nutr Metab 2016;41(9):1002–4.
40. Lis D, Ahuja KD, Stellingwerff T, et al. Case study: utilizing a low FODMAP diet to combat exercise-induced gastrointestinal symptoms. Int J Sport Nutr Exerc Metab 2016;26(5):481–7.
41. DeFilippis EM, Tabani S, Warren RU, et al. Exercise and self-reported limitations in patients with inflammatory bowel disease. Dig Dis Sci 2016;61(1):215–20.
42. Orchard TR. Management of arthritis in patients with inflammatory bowel disease. Gastroenterol Hepatol (N Y) 2012;8(5):327–9.
43. Bilski J, Mazur-Bialy A, Brzozowski B, et al. Can exercise affect the course of inflammatory bowel disease? Experimental and clinical evidence. Pharmacol Rep 2016;68(4):827–36.
44. Bilski J, Brzozowski B, Mazur-Bialy A, et al. The role of physical exercise in inflammatory bowel disease. Biomed Res Int 2014;2014:429031.
45. Ploeger H, Obeid J, Nguyen T, et al. Exercise and inflammation in pediatric Crohn's disease. Int J Sports Med 2012;33(8):671–9.

46. Rosenblatt E, Kane S. Sex-specific issues in inflammatory bowel disease. Gastroenterol Hepatol (N Y) 2015;11(9):592–601.
47. Lucak S, Chang L, Halpert A, et al. Current and emergent pharmacologic treatments for irritable bowel syndrome with diarrhea: evidence-based treatment in practice. Therap Adv Gastroenterol 2017;10(2):253–75.
48. Payne S. Sex, gender, and irritable bowel syndrome: making the connections. Gend Med 2004;1(1):18–28.
49. Chey WD, Kurlander J, Eswaran S. Irritable bowel syndrome: a clinical review. JAMA 2015;313(9):949–58.
50. Bird ST, Liu W, Brophy JM, et al. Irritable bowel syndrome and drospirenone-containing oral contraceptives; a comparative-safety study. Curr Drug Saf 2012;7(1):8–15.
51. Sebastian Domingo JJ. The new Rome criteria (IV) of functional digestive disorders in clinical practice. Med Clin (Barc) 2017. http://dx.doi.org/10.1016/j.medcli.2016.12.020.
52. Menees SB, Powell C, Kurlander J, et al. A meta-analysis of the utility of C-reactive protein, erythrocyte sedimentation rate, fecal calprotectin, and fecal lactoferrin to exclude inflammatory bowel disease in adults with IBS. Am J Gastroenterol 2015;110(3):444–54.
53. Cronin O, O'Sullivan O, Barton W, et al. Gut microbiota: implications for sports and exercise medicine. Br J Sports Med 2017;51(9):700–1.
54. Daley AJ, Grimmett C, Roberts L, et al. The effects of exercise upon symptoms and quality of life in patients diagnosed with irritable bowel syndrome: a randomised controlled trial. Int J Sports Med 2008;29(9):778–82.
55. Johannesson E, Simren M, Strid H, et al. Physical activity improves symptoms in irritable bowel syndrome: a randomized controlled trial. Am J Gastroenterol 2011; 106(5):915–22.

Female Athlete Triad

Future Directions for Energy Availability and Eating Disorder Research and Practice

Nancy I. Williams, ScD[a],*, Siobhan M. Statuta, MD[b], Ashley Austin, MD[b]

KEYWORDS

- Low energy availability • Eating disorders • Female • Athlete • Exercise
- Female Athlete Triad

KEY POINTS

- The impact of low energy availability (EA) on reproductive function can be modified by gynecologic age, psychological factors, and genetics. As such, a more individualized approach to diagnosing and treating low EA is warranted.
- In practice, the accurate measurement of EA (in combination with the difficulties of diagnosing and treating the increasing number of athletes with disordered eating) represent key challenges in Triad research going forward.
- Recently published guidelines for determining Triad risk stratification, including guidance for clearance and return to play, represent a critical step in the advancement of evidence-based translation, but need to be refined and validated moving forward. It is critical that sports medicine practitioners and researchers work together to achieve this goal, which, in turn, will more effectively reduce the prevalence of the Female Athlete Triad.

INTRODUCTION

In the 1990s, the concept of the Female Athlete Triad was introduced, drawing attention to a syndrome of 3 tightly interrelated conditions: disordered eating (DE), amenorrhea, and osteoporosis.[1] The definition of the Triad was revised in 2007 to its current meaning to include 1 or more of the following 3 components:

1. Low energy availability (EA) (with or without DE)
2. Menstrual dysfunction
3. Low bone mineral density (BMD)

Disclosure Statements: N.I. Williams has nothing to disclose.
[a] Noll Laboratory, Department of Kinesiology, Women's Health and Exercise Laboratories, Penn State University, Room 108, University Park, PA 16802, USA; [b] Department of Family Medicine, University of Virginia Health System, PO Box 800729, Charlottesville, VA 22908, USA
* Corresponding author.
E-mail address: niw1@psu.edu

Clin Sports Med 36 (2017) 671–686
http://dx.doi.org/10.1016/j.csm.2017.05.003
0278-5919/17/© 2017 Elsevier Inc. All rights reserved.

This also includes the continuum between healthy and unhealthy states for each of the 3 elements.[2] Several seminal studies in the 1980s[3–5] piqued the interest of clinicians and researchers alike, and almost 4 decades of research now serves as the foundation for our understanding of this complex medical condition. The existence of the Triad is widespread, with prevalence varying by sport. Sports that demand high energy expenditure, a lean physique, and/or an aesthetic component carry the greatest incidence.[6] The clinical, behavioral, and physiologic consequences of the Triad are extensive and include clinical eating disorders and DE, osteopenia, transient infertility, dyslipidemia, impaired endothelial function,[7–9] performance-related issues such as stress fractures,[10–12] fatigue, and decrements in competitive performance.[13] Much progress has been made in our understanding of the underlying behaviors and physiology of these conditions,[14–16] as well as the creation of practical recommendations for prevention, screening, treatment, and return to play.[2,17,18] However, many gaps still exist in the literature and in the translation of research into practice. The purpose of this article is to highlight future potential directions for research by drawing attention to areas in the Triad literature that require clarification. From there, these data may be applied to the clinical setting for more evidence-supported interventions. For recent reviews on the Female Athlete Triad, the reader is referred to other sources.[19–24]

LOW ENERGY AVAILABILITY: GAPS AND CLARIFICATIONS

EA has been a focus of Triad research since the 2007 American College of Sports Medicine Position Stand[2] on the Female Athlete Triad emphasized the critical role of EA (with or without DE) in the etiology of the Triad. Current knowledge on the underlying mechanism of exercise-related menstrual disorders has been informed by prospective studies in nonhuman primates[25] and previously untrained women.[3,26] These have shown that aerobic exercise, in combination with caloric restriction, can induce menstrual disturbances. Menstrual function is restored when energy intake (EI) (and, in turn, EA) is increased during periods of exercise. This demonstrates a causal role of low EA in the induction and the vital role it plays in the reversal of exercise-associated menstrual disturbances.[25,27] EA also plays an important role in maintaining skeletal health in exercising women. This is evidenced by its association with altered bone parameters independent of estrogen status,[28,29] and by the dysregulation of important bone-related hormones when Triad conditions are present.[30–33]

Although the causal role of low EA in the development of Triad conditions is well supported, several issues deserve consideration. The elegant studies of Loucks and colleagues[34] are frequently cited to support a particular calculation of EA that represents the difference between the total calories consumed as food and the caloric expenditure of exercise, normalized for fat-free mass (ffm).

$$\frac{(\text{daily dietary intake (kcals)} - \text{daily exercise energy expenditure (kcals)})}{\text{ffm (kg)}}$$

Short-term (5-day) reductions in EA below a threshold of 30 kcal/kg ffm per day have been found to slow the normal pulsatile release of luteinizing hormone (LH) from the anterior pituitary gland, a proxy indicator of hypothalamic gonadotropic-releasing hormone (GnRH) secretion.[35] A slowing of LH pulse frequency is, in turn, associated with delays in folliculogenesis, luteal phase shortening, and more severe menstrual disturbances.[25,36–38] This reduced LH pulse frequency occurs regardless of whether EA is reduced via diet, exercise, or a combination of the two.[34] When EA is considered to be the energy required to support a body's basic physiologic processes, it becomes clear that effects will be extensive as levels decline. Specifically, once EA is reduced below the 30 kcal/kg ffm per day threshold mentioned previously, some of the observed metabolic alterations include reduced serum concentrations of glucose, triiodothyronine, insulin, insulinlike growth factor-1, and elevations in growth hormone and cortisol.[34,35]

The previous studies demonstrate the importance of EA in the modulation of LH pulse frequency with reductions associated with subclinical menstrual disturbances[39,40] and amenorrhea.[41,42] Yet, much more needs to be clarified to further our understanding. For example, the precise magnitude of reduction in EA, or rather, the degree of energy deficit associated with the initial disruption of ovarian function has not been directly demonstrated through experimentation. Although we know an EA below the threshold of 30 kcal/kg ffm per day modifies LH pulsatility and metabolism, we do not know what magnitude of change in LH pulsatile dynamics is associated with the induction of menstrual disturbances, as this has not been prospectively evaluated in humans. In a recent randomized trial, Williams and colleagues[26] demonstrated that luteal phase defects, oligomenorrhea, and anovulation were induced by energy deficits ranging from −22% to −42% of baseline energy needs (−470 kcal to −810 kcal below initial energy requirements). These outcomes provide practical information about the magnitude of caloric deficiency resulting in exercise-associated menstrual disturbances. However, the assessment of actual energy balance is difficult and expensive to calculate. Furthermore, it varies significantly as it adjusts in attempts to conserve energy, restore energy balance, and stabilize weight.[43] As such, future studies should address the magnitude of change in EA as calculated by Loucks and colleagues[44] that is associated with the induction of menstrual disturbances. To that end, a preliminary report by Leiberman and colleagues[45] demonstrates that EA is linearly related to the risk of menstrual disturbances and that no clear threshold below which ovarian function is disrupted exists. Rather, as EA drops below 30 kcal · ffm^{-1}, the risk of a menstrual disturbance increases above 50%. Regardless of the level of EA at which reproductive function is disrupted, current recommendations[46] to maintain EA at approximately 45 kcal · ffm^{-1} are supported. It is clear, however, that a need exists for additional research regarding energy thresholds as well as the identification of easier, less expensive methods to calculate energy deficits.

One future research area to prioritize includes the validation of repeated assessments using field measures of EA that accurately reflect the EA calculations of Loucks, and colleagues.[44] These calculations could additionally be used to explore new methods of monitoring energy status such as repeated measurements of body mass index (BMI), weight loss, and percent body fat. Traditionally, these data have been difficult to interpret given the variability of the Triad athlete presentations. For example, a single measurement of body weight and/or BMI may reveal overt undernutrition and chronic energy deficiency if values are less than 85% of expected body weight, BMI less than 17.5 kg m^2, or if an adolescent's BMI is <50th percentile.[43] However, if these measures do not reveal an energy deficit, additional, more reliable measures are required to determine low EA. The ideal biomarker of energy status would be one that can be accurately and objectively measured to scale and is reflective of compensatory adaptations to chronic energy deficiency (ie, body weight can remain stable even when EA is low). Furthermore, to enhance its applicability, the biomarker would need to be reflective of changes in EA over the same time frame that is associated with changes in ovarian function. One such biomarker, triiodothyronine, may fit these criteria. Because body weight stability can be observed despite a low EA state,[44] physiologic signs of energy conservation should be assessed, such as blood concentrations of total triiodothyronine and measures of the ratio of actual to predicted resting metabolic rate.[17] Future studies would ideally determine the reliability and validity of any EA biomarker.

As noted previously, the current lack of reproducibility in the methods of assessing energy deficiency has limited the widespread implementation of EA assessments. Another potential approach to diagnosing low EA is to target the more qualitative assessment of eating behaviors and attitudes to identify the factors related to the underconsumption of energy relative to energy expenditure. This may be an alternative approach to quantifying energy intake and/or energy expenditure in athletes who are underconsuming food due to conscious restriction. In support of this, studies have documented significant associations between drive for thinness, cognitive restraint, and EA.[47,48] Regardless of the approach, it is important that any measurements demonstrate acceptable levels of sensitivity and specificity if particular cutoffs for indicators of EA are used in decision-making rules for individual athletes. A recent review by Joy and colleagues[49] provides very useful information regarding the clinical assessment and management of eating disorders (ED) and DE in athletes on which future studies can expand.

ETIOLOGY OF LOW ENERGY AVAILABILITY

Appropriate treatment of low EA as it relates to the induction of menstrual and bone sequelae requires an understanding of how and why EA is low. What is the pathway to low EA? As described in the Female Athlete Triad Coalition Consensus Statement,[43] there are 4 distinct pathways to low EA:

- DE
- Clinical eating disorder (ED)
- Intentional weight loss without DE
- Inadvertent undereating

As such, screening and treatment strategies need to target these individual pathways. If the etiology of low EA involves DE, medical attention and nutrition education are warranted. A clinical ED should trigger medical, psychological, and nutritional education interventions, each with monitored components. Similarly, weight loss without DE also should involve nutritional education. A less well understood basis for low EA is inadvertent undereating, which presumably occurs when caloric intake does not meet energy expenditure needs in the absence of conscious restriction of food intake. The extent to which inadvertent undereating contributes to the Triad is currently unclear. Possible explanations for inadvertent undereating could include practical and logistic challenges, such as access to and/or affordability of food and beverages. Unfortunately, the prevalence of these issues has not been well documented. The physiologic suppression of hunger in response to the intensity or volume of exercise has been demonstrated in prospective studies and therefore appetite is not considered a reliable indicator of energy requirements in endurance sports.[44,50,51] There exist many questions regarding inadvertent undereating, as there are not much data available. In fact, most studies of female athletes with Triad conditions provide evidence of DE in the form of body image disturbances, measures of restrictive food intake, or pathogenic weight control behaviors in association with menstrual disturbances and low bone mass.[14,52,53] A recent report on the prevalence of individual and combined Triad conditions from more than 65 studies found that the prevalence of clinical ED and DE ranged from 0% to 48% and 7.1% to 89.2%, respectively. Future studies need to document the extent to which, and the mechanisms whereby, inadvertent undereating contributes to low EA associated with the Triad.

GYNECOLOGIC AGE

The importance of low EA as a causal factor in Triad conditions has been established. Yet, the individual variation in the susceptibility to low EA may be attributable to factors that modify the relation among EA, ovarian disruption, and/or bone metabolism. A critical factor that has not been addressed in Triad literature is gynecologic age; that is, the difference between one's chronologic age and the age of menarche. The natural prevalence of menstrual disturbances decreases with advancing age until the time of perimenopause.[54] In a variety of species, the impact of various stressors on the reproductive axis also decreases as reproductive opportunity decreases.[55] Evidence for the effects of gynecologic age were reported by Loucks,[56] who showed that decreases in LH pulsatility caused by low EA (EA <10 kcal/kg ffm), were dependent on gynecologic age. They noted that subjects whose gynecologic age ranged from 14 to 18 years did not experience a decrease in LH pulse frequency, whereas those with a gynecologic age of 5 to 8 years did. Gynecologic maturity was also cited as a factor in the prospective 12-month marathon training study by Rogol and colleagues[57] who reported that no significant changes occurred in any LH pulse parameter in women who were 17.8 ± 0.9 years post menarche. However, this study was criticized because the exercising women began the intervention with some indications of exercise-induced menstrual disturbances at the outset, which may have prevented the ability to see the effects of the year-long training.[58] In a prospective study composed of women aged 25 to 40 years who participated in an exercise training program combined with caloric restriction to achieve modest weight loss, few disruptions in menstrual regularity occurred.[59] Taken together, these studies indicate that the risk of developing menstrual disturbances in association with exercise may decline with advanced gynecologic age. This is an important translational finding, as practitioners should take gynecologic age into account when assessing the risk of exercise-associated menstrual disturbances and determining the need for Female Athlete Triad prevention strategies in gynecologically mature athletes.

GENETICS

An individual's genetics may contribute to one's susceptibility to functional hypothalamic amenorrhea (FHA). Caronia and colleagues[60] reported that in a sample of 55 women with FHA, 7 had heterozygous mutations associated with hypothalamic hypogonadism, in which mutations to the following genes were found: fibroblast growth factor receptor-1, the Kallmann syndrome 1 sequence, prokineticin receptor 2, and the GnRH receptor. No such mutations were found in 422 control subjects with normal menstrual cycles. Each of the affected genes serve unique and significant roles. The Kallmann syndrome 1 sequence gene and the prokineticin receptor 2 gene both play a key role in the migration of GnRH-secreting neurons.[61,62] The fibroblast growth factor receptor-1 gene determines differentiation, migration, and maintenance of GnRH secreting neurons.[63] Last, the GnRH receptor gene encodes the receptor that GnRH binds to on the gonadotrophs.[64] Consequently, individuals with FHA may possess defects important to GnRH secretion and regulation, therefore making their hypothalamic pituitary ovarian function vulnerable to stress-induced dysfunction (ie, low EA). More research is necessary to determine the extent to which genetic factors may contribute to menstrual cycle disturbances in exercising women of all ages.

PSYCHOLOGICAL FACTORS

Although much of the Triad condition relates to states of low EA, it is well documented that psychological and social stress can impact reproductive function in humans and animals.[65–73] Despite this fact, specific Triad literature lacks the recognition that exercise-associated menstrual disturbances are a subtype of this stress-induced reproductive disruption paralleling anorexia, DE, bulimia, and other psychosocial stressors. It is likely that these exercise-induced menstrual disturbances involve elements of psychosocial stress, as metabolic and psychosocial stressors coexist in everyday life and are difficult to tease apart. Even though clinical eating disorders, such as anorexia and bulimia, are considered stress-related disorders, the singular focus on the energy availability aspects of these psychiatric disorders as the primary mechanism underlying reproductive dysfunction ignores the potential contribution of additional suppressive effects of neuroendocrine pathways associated with psychogenic factors against a background of energy deficiency. In fact, synergistic effects of a combination of metabolic and psychosocial stressors on the disruption of menstrual function have been demonstrated in a monkey model.[74] Bethea and colleagues[75,76] extended these findings to show that individual differences in stress sensitivity to the aforementioned multistress paradigm are associated with alterations in central neurotransmitter systems.

Similar to these animal experiments, additional studies in humans have demonstrated that women with FHA have psychological phenotypes suggestive of high stress responsiveness.[77,78] These women commonly display dysfunctional attitudes, difficulty coping with daily hassles, a higher dependence on interpersonal relationships, higher incidence of past psychiatric disorders, and subclinical symptoms of depression and anxiety. A randomized controlled trial using cognitive behavioral therapy to treat the aforementioned abnormal psychological profiles in women with FHA demonstrated that women who received the therapy had an ovarian recovery rate of 87.5% versus a 25.0% recovery rate in the control group that received no treatment.[79] A follow-up study detailed the neuroendocrine changes that accompanied the recovery of ovarian function.[80] To highlight the importance of psychosocial change in the recovery of ovarian function, it is important to note that the work by Berga and colleagues[79] represented exercising women with menstrual disturbances who continued to exercise as a part of therapy in addition to using behavioral change techniques to make healthy adjustments to dietary intake.

The mechanism underlying the effects of psychosocial stressors on menstrual function is commonly thought to be the stress-induced activation of the hypothalamic-pituitary-adrenal axis,[81] but the actual neuroendocrine mechanisms that suppress GnRH neuronal activity remain unclear.[82–84] A challenging aspect in identifying these mechanisms is that psychogenic stressors are often associated with metabolic stress because food intake is reduced. In many stress studies, this is overlooked, as food intake and body weight changes are often not quantified or reported. Loucks and Redman[85] have explored this conundrum, concluding that the underlying mechanism whereby psychogenic stressors act to suppress the reproductive axis is through their impact on energy balance. The challenge of teasing out psychogenic versus metabolic factors associated with menstrual disturbances in exercising women has also been addressed.[86,87] Future research should comprehensively examine the role of psychosocial factors in the development and reversal of Triad conditions.

Given the complexity of how the key role of low EA in the etiology of menstrual disturbances may be modified by factors such as gynecologic age, genetics, and psychogenic stress, it is important that future research explores the relative importance of these effects. Other fertile areas for research include the impact of racial and cultural differences on an individual's susceptibility to stress-induced reproductive disturbances. Although progress has occurred regarding the application of research findings to the development of recommendations for athletes and sports medicine practitioners, the move toward more "precise" and "personalized" medicine should foster evidence-based approaches to Triad prevention and treatments that incorporate a more comprehensive understanding of physiologic and psychosocial influences on menstrual function and/or bone metabolism.

FEMALE ATHLETE TRIAD AND RELATIVE ENERGY DEFICIENCY IN SPORT

As Triad research evolves, it is important to keep in focus that the primary physiologic and clinical presentations of the Triad continue to be low EA with or without DE, menstrual disturbances, and low bone mass. These are the medical conditions that clinicians and practitioners have deemed clinically important enough to warrant treatment and prevention strategies. Secondary physiologic and clinical consequences of the Triad have also been documented in exercising women, including alterations in metabolism,[88–91] lipid profiles,[8,92] cardiovascular function,[92–94] and bone stress injury.[95,96] These changes are mechanistically linked to the Triad related to the chronic hypoestrogenic state and long-term low EA.[95] Recently, the International Olympic Committee (IOC) described their version of this concept of low EA in the acronym "RED-S" or "relative energy deficiency in sport." They emphasize a broader impact that low EA may have on additional physiologic systems outside of the hypothalamic pituitary gonadal axis and bone.[97] The juxtaposition of this recent IOC statement with existing Triad literature has generated debate and confusion.[18,98,99] The investigators propose that "relative energy deficiency" (which is not quantitatively defined) is a common problem for both female and male individuals in sport, and that its effects are widespread across a variety of organ systems.[97] The RED-S concept broadly considers all bodily processes that may be affected by relative energy deficiency equally and depicts the relation between low EA and each aspect of physiology as a direct association. In contrast, previous research and position stands on the Triad have repeatedly documented specific physiologic effects associated with low EA[2,95] (ie, alterations in metabolic hormones) and those associated with clinical eating disorders (ie, gastrointestinal [GI] disturbances). These outcomes represent part of the primary underlying mechanism of energy conservation (as in the case of hormonal changes), as well as the secondary disturbances (the GI disturbances) in relation to the principal components of the Female Athlete Triad. Notably, the prevalence, severity, and clinical importance of secondary effects of chronic low EA, such as those seen in immune and vascular function, have not yet been irrefutably established. In the meantime, clinicians and practitioners should not lose sight of the established clinical importance and treatment recommendations associated with the Female Athlete Triad as more data regarding other body systems are explored. Future research should include direct comparisons of the validity of approaches used for risk stratification, treatment, and return to play in recent consensus statements.[43,97] More research on the effects of low EA in male individuals, individuals of different abilities, and individuals from different racial backgrounds is highlighted by Mountjoy and colleagues.[97]

MALE ATHLETE TRIAD

Interest in whether a parallel to the Female Athlete Triad occurs in male athletes has increased recently.[100] Clinically, this is a challenge to ascertain, as outward reproductive manifestations are difficult to identify and may require sperm and fertility testing as well as tracking of hormone levels. Testosterone levels are affected by physical activity with levels shifting in response to time/duration of exercise, endurance versus resistance-trained sport, and age.[101] Testosterone production can also decrease in overtraining or conditions of decreased EA.[102] Manifestations on bone health are less clear, as available studies have been in small samples across varying ages and sports. For endurance athletes, levels of sex hormones tend to be reduced,[103] and values outside of the normal range have been associated with impaired bone health.[100] However, Ackerman and colleagues[104] showed that levels of estradiol were positively correlated with higher BMD, raising questions regarding the possible effects of estradiol on bone health in male individuals beyond that of the classically considered testosterone. Currently, parallels between male and female athletes in low energy conditions are being further examined. There clearly exists a dearth of information, requiring further research in areas such as nutritional deficits in male athletes and vitamin supplementation with regard to bone health. Applying conclusions found in the female population to male individuals is not substantiated, and caution should be encouraged. Future research should highlight the magnitude of change in EA that is associated with clinical and physiologic sequelae in both reproductive and bone health outcomes in male athletes, especially considering that it may prove to be different from what has been found in female athletes.

EATING DISORDERS AND DISORDERED EATING

Most cases of the Female Athlete Triad involve low EA that results from the conscious restriction of food intake that occurs along a continuum of severity. As Joy and colleagues[49] noted in a recent extensive review, the concern surrounding eating behaviors in athletes is pressing, as the rates of EDs in the general population are on the rise for individuals in their late teenage years[105] and are high among elite adolescent athletes.[106] Added attention to certain research gaps would assist with demystifying this entity and would allow for earlier identification of potential problematic athlete cases, as this is thought to be crucial for the recovery process.[107] There exists no simple method for detection of EDs, and although questionnaires exist, studies indicate that a clinical interview is the best option among elite athletes and controls.[106] More recent screening approaches that complement established ED inventories[108,109] or interview strategies[110] includes the Brief ED in Athletes Questionnaire (BEDA-Q).[111] An alternative is the LEAF-Q (Low Energy Availability in Females Questionnaire), which has been shown to predict overall Triad risk independent of whether DE is present.[112] Future studies should continue to focus on fast and accurate ways to screen and diagnose DE/ED in female athletes with attention toward the effectiveness of these approaches on an individual basis. Regarding the specificity of methodological approaches, the review by Bratland-Sanda and Sundgot-Borgen effectively points out that previously proposed risk factors need to be scientifically validated by showing a clear, causal relationship through more prospective, large-scale, and longer-term studies.[113] There also exists a need for an extensive literature review of general, as well as more specific, risk factors across sport and gender including weight cycling and dieting pressures, personality traits, early sport specialization, history of injury, and sport regulations (especially in those emphasizing leanness).[113] Suggested risk factors need to be scientifically validated by showing a cause-and-effect relationship. By having a more sport specific checklist of confirmed items to watch for, a more timely recognition and management process can be initiated.[113] Besides refining the checklist of risk factors and improving diagnosis, intervening through education shows potential value in the prevention of eating pathologies. Recent advancements regarding educational interventions targeting adolescent athletes and coaches to prevent the development of ED[114,115] should be a focus going forward.

Another area of potential investigative focus is the clarification of when an athlete identified to be on the ED-DE spectrum is too ill for sport participation. How soon will the recovering athlete be well enough to resume sport, and to what degree? These are clinical conundrums encountered regularly without any clear or applicable consensus. The current consensus statements are beneficial but do not address specifics as basic as warranted exercise limitations on identification of an ED. Delineation of more explicit sport-specific guidelines would offer invaluable guidance to those health care providers overseeing athlete recovery and safe guidance back into sport. Similarly, completion of a simple yet thorough review of current clinical practices by these care providers would provide applicable and real-life data to help identify the direction of future position statements/guidelines. A review would also help in refining previously published strategies for Triad risk stratification.[43] With actual data illustrating the real-world clinical successes and hurdles, providers and care teams can focus on more efficient and practical approaches to the athlete.

APPLYING TRIAD SCIENCE AND CLINICAL JUDGMENT TO INFORM CLEARANCE AND RETURN TO PLAY DECISIONS

Although the scientific underpinnings and epidemiology of the Female Athlete Triad have been well explored in the literature and updated position stands are available, a gap in practice-based applications of Triad science still exists. This is arguably the most difficult step in addressing public health issues, and as such, represents a gap in the area of the Female Athlete Triad. The recent Female Athlete Triad Coalition Consensus Statement[43] provided the first comprehensive effort to provide clinicians and practitioners with recommendations for clearing athletes for competition and returning them to play. As a joint effort among leading scientists, physicians, nutritionists, and other sports medicine experts, the statement advances the field of Triad research because it provides an evidence-based approach to risk stratification, including an easy to use algorithm for incorporating Triad-related risk factors into decision-making processes for clearance and return to play of individual athletes. Another approach, "Red Light, Yellow Light, Green Light," has been developed and is described by Mountjoy and colleagues.[97] These guidelines are based on scientific evidence and must be used in the context of clinical judgment while considering "decision modifiers," such as the type of sport, the timing during the season, the position played, and so forth. These approaches represent the translation of Triad science into practice at an organizational and policy level, with recent reports confirming that these recommendations are being implemented and adapted.[116,117] Future research should include refinements and modifications to these algorithms that improve their sensitivity and specificity.

SUMMARY

Research on the Female Athlete Triad has spanned several decades. Despite this, there still exist many gaps in the research. Low EA is the key factor in the etiology of the Triad, but the impact of low EA on reproductive function can be modified by gynecologic age, psychological factors, genetics, and likely many other factors. As such, a more individualized approach to diagnosing and treating low EA is warranted, and more research is necessary to improve the measurement of EA and how these measurements are incorporated into decisions regarding clearance and return to play. The difficulties of diagnosing and treating the increasing number of athletes with DE also represent key challenges in Triad research going forward. Screening instruments that are validated for use in individual athletes are needed, as are effective educational and behavioral interventions applied to both coaches and athletes for the prevention and treatment of ED and DE. Recently published guidelines for determining Triad risk stratification and providing guidance for clearance and return to play represent a critical step in the advancement of an evidence-based translation and need to be refined and validated going forward. It is critical that sports medicine practitioners and researchers continue to work together with these challenges in mind to achieve the goal of reducing the prevalence of the Female Athlete Triad.

REFERENCES

1. Otis CL, Drinkwater B, Johnson M, et al. American College of Sports Medicine position stand. The female athlete triad. Med Sci Sports Exerc 1997;29(5):i–ix.
2. Nattiv A, Loucks AB, Manore MM, et al. American College of Sports Medicine position stand. The female athlete triad. Med Sci Sports Exerc 2007;39(10): 1867–82.
3. Bullen BA, Skrinar GS, Beitins IZ, et al. Induction of menstrual disorders by strenuous exercise in untrained women. N Engl J Med 1985;312(21):1349–53.
4. Drinkwater BL, Nilson K, Chesnut CH 3rd, et al. Bone mineral content of amenorrheic and eumenorrheic athletes. N Engl J Med 1984;311(5):277–81.
5. Brooks-Gunn J, Warren MP, Hamilton LH. The relation of eating problems and amenorrhea in ballet dancers. Med Sci Sports Exerc 1987;19(1):41–4.
6. Torstveit MK, Sundgot-Borgen J. The female athlete triad: are elite athletes at increased risk? Med Sci Sports Exerc 2005;37(2):184–93.
7. Hoch AZ, Jurva JW, Staton MA, et al. Athletic amenorrhea and endothelial dysfunction. WMJ 2007;106(6):301–6.
8. Friday KE, Drinkwater BL, Bruemmer B, et al. Elevated plasma low-density lipoprotein and high-density lipoprotein cholesterol levels in amenorrheic athletes: effects of endogenous hormone status and nutrient intake. J Clin Endocrinol Metab 1993;77(6):1605–9.
9. O'Donnell E, De Souza MJ. The cardiovascular effects of chronic hypoestrogenism in amenorrhoeic athletes: a critical review. Sports Med 2004;34(9):601–27.
10. Bennell K, Matheson G, Meeuwisse W, et al. Risk factors for stress fractures. Sports Med 1999;28(2):91–122.
11. Barrow GW, Saha S. Menstrual irregularity and stress-fractures in collegiate female distance runners. Am J Sports Med 1988;16(3):209–16.
12. Brukner P, Bennell K. Stress fractures in female athletes—diagnosis, management and rehabilitation. Sports Med 1997;24(6):419–29.
13. Vanheest JL, Rodgers CD, Mahoney CE, et al. Ovarian suppression impairs sport performance in junior elite female swimmers. Med Sci Sports Exerc 2014;46(1):156–66.
14. Gibbs JC, Williams NI, De Souza MJ. Prevalence of individual and combined components of the female athlete triad. Med Sci Sports Exerc 2013;45(5): 985–96.
15. Sundgot-Borgen J, Torstveit MK. Prevalence of eating disorders in elite athletes is higher than in the general population. Clin J Sport Med 2004;14(1):25–32.
16. Nichols JF, Rauh MJ, Lawson MJ, et al. Prevalence of the female athlete triad syndrome among high school athletes. Arch Pediatr Adolesc Med 2006; 160(2):137–42.
17. De Souza MJ, Nattiv A, Joy E, et al. 2014 female athlete triad coalition consensus statement on treatment and return to play of the female athlete triad: 1st International Conference held in San Francisco, CA, May 2012, and 2nd International Conference held in Indianapolis, IN, May 2013. Clin J Sport Med 2014;24(2):96–119.

18. De Souza MJ, Williams NI, Nattiv A, et al. Misunderstanding the female athlete triad: refuting the IOC consensus statement on relative energy deficiency in sport (RED-S). Br J Sports Med 2014;48(20):1461–5.
19. Thein-Nissenbaum J. Long term consequences of the female athlete triad. Maturitas 2013;75(2):107–12.
20. Thein-Nissenbaum JM, Carr KE. Female athlete triad syndrome in the high school athlete. Phys Ther Sport 2011;12(3):108–16.
21. Matzkin E, Curry EJ, Whitlock K. Female athlete triad: past, present, and future. J Am Acad Orthop Surg 2015;23(7):424–32.
22. Javed A, Tebben PJ, Fischer PR, et al. Female athlete triad and its components: toward improved screening and management. Mayo Clin Proc 2013;88(9): 996–1009.
23. Hergenroeder AC, De Souza MJ, Anding RH. The female athlete triad: energy deficiency, physiologic consequences, and treatment. Adolesc Med State Art Rev 2015;26(1):116–42.
24. Barrack MT, Ackerman KE, Gibbs JC. Update on the female athlete triad. Curr Rev Musculoskelet Med 2013;6(2):195–204.
25. Williams NI, Helmreich DL, Parfitt DB, et al. Evidence for a causal role of low energy availability in the induction of menstrual cycle disturbances during strenuous exercise training. J Clin Endocrinol Metab 2001;86(11):5184–93.
26. Williams NI, Leidy HJ, Hill BR, et al. Magnitude of daily energy deficit predicts frequency but not severity of menstrual disturbances associated with exercise and caloric restriction. Am J Physiol Endocrinol Metab 2015;308(1):E29–39.
27. Kopp-Woodroffe SA, Manore MM, Dueck CA, et al. Energy and nutrient status of amenorrheic athletes participating in a diet and exercise training intervention program. Int J Sport Nutr 1999;9(1):70–88.
28. De Souza MJ, West SL, Jamal SA, et al. The presence of both an energy deficiency and estrogen deficiency exacerbate alterations of bone metabolism in exercising women. Bone 2008;43(1):140–8.
29. Southmayd EA, Mallinson RJ, Williams NI, et al. Unique effects of energy versus estrogen deficiency on multiple components of bone strength in exercising women. Osteoporos Int 2017;28(4):1365–76.
30. Ihle R, Loucks AB. Dose-response relationships between energy availability and bone turnover in young exercising women. J Bone Miner Res 2004;19(8): 1231–40.
31. Hilton LK, Loucks AB. Low energy availability, not exercise stress, suppresses the diurnal rhythm of leptin in healthy young women. Am J Physiol Endocrinol Metab 2000;278(1):E43–9.
32. Loucks AB, Mortola JF, Girton L, et al. Alterations in the hypothalamic-pituitary-ovarian and the hypothalamic-pituitary-adrenal axes in athletic women. J Clin Endocrinol Metab 1989;68(2):402–11.
33. Misra M, Klibanski A. Bone health in anorexia nervosa. Curr Opin Endocrinol Diabetes Obes 2011;18(6):376–82.
34. Loucks AB, Verdun M, Heath EM. Low energy availability, not stress of exercise, alters LH pulsatility in exercising women. J Appl Physiol 1998;84(1):37–46.
35. Loucks AB, Thuma JR. Luteinizing hormone pulsatility is disrupted at a threshold of energy availability in regularly menstruating women. J Clin Endocrinol Metab 2003;88(1):297–311.
36. Lucy MC, Staples CR, Michel FM, et al. Energy balance and size and number of ovarian follicles detected by ultrasonography in early postpartum dairy cows. J Dairy Sci 1991;74(2):473–82.

37. Murphy MG, Enright WJ, Crowe MA, et al. Effect of dietary intake on pattern of growth of dominant follicles during the oestrous cycle in beef heifers. J Reprod Fertil 1991;92(2):333–8.

38. Knobil E. The neuroendocrine control of the menstrual cycle. Recent Prog Horm Res 1980;36:53–88.

39. Filicori M, Flamigni C, Campaniello E, et al. Evidence for a specific role of GnRH pulse frequency in the control of the human menstrual cycle. Am J Physiol 1989; 257(6 Pt 1):E930–6.

40. Soules MR, Clifton DK, Cohen NL, et al. Luteal phase deficiency: abnormal gonadotropin and progesterone secretion patterns. J Clin Endocrinol Metab 1989;69(4):813–20.

41. Filicori M, Tabarelli C, Casadio P, et al. Interaction between menstrual cyclicity and gonadotropin pulsatility. Horm Res 1998;49(3–4):169–72.

42. Santoro N, Filicori M, Crowley WF Jr. Hypogonadotropic disorders in men and women: diagnosis and therapy with pulsatile gonadotropin-releasing hormone. Endocr Rev 1986;7(1):11–23.

43. De Souza MJ, Nattiv A, Joy E, et al. 2014 female athlete triad coalition consensus statement on treatment and return to play of the female athlete triad: 1st International Conference held in San Francisco, California, May 2012 and 2nd International Conference held in Indianapolis, Indiana, May 2013. Br J Sports Med 2014;48(4):289.

44. Loucks AB, Kiens B, Wright HH. Energy availability in athletes. J Sports Sci 2011;29(Suppl 1):S7–15.

45. Leiberman JL, De Souza MJ, Williams NI. Luteal phase defects induced by exercise and diet are associated with low energy availability. Med Sci Sports Exerc 2013;45(S5):520–1.

46. Joy E, De Souza MJ, Nattiv A, et al. 2014 female athlete triad coalition consensus statement on treatment and return to play of the female athlete triad. Curr Sports Med Rep 2014;13(4):219–32.

47. Gibbs JC, Williams NI, Mallinson RJ, et al. Effect of high dietary restraint on energy availability and menstrual status. Med Sci Sports Exerc 2013;45(9):1790–7.

48. Gibbs JC, Williams NI, Scheid JL, et al. The association of a high drive for thinness with energy deficiency and severe menstrual disturbances: confirmation in a large population of exercising women. Int J Sport Nutr Exerc Metab 2011; 21(4):280–90.

49. Joy E, Kussman A, Nattiv A. 2016 update on eating disorders in athletes: a comprehensive narrative review with a focus on clinical assessment and management. Br J Sports Med 2016;50(3):154–62.

50. Stubbs RJ, Sepp A, Hughes DA, et al. The effect of graded levels of exercise on energy intake and balance in free-living women. Int J Obes Relat Metab Disord 2002;26(6):866–9.

51. Whybrow S, Hughes DA, Ritz P, et al. The effect of an incremental increase in exercise on appetite, eating behaviour and energy balance in lean men and women feeding ad libitum. Br J Nutr 2008;100(5):1109–15.

52. Thein-Nissenbaum JM, Rauh MJ, Carr KE, et al. Associations between disordered eating, menstrual dysfunction, and musculoskeletal injury among high school athletes. J Orthop Sports Phys Ther 2011;41(2):60–9.

53. Rauh MJ, Nichols JF, Barrack MT. Relationships among injury and disordered eating, menstrual dysfunction, and low bone mineral density in high school athletes: a prospective study. J Athl Train 2010;45(3):243–52.

54. Hambridge HL, Mumford SL, Mattison DR, et al. The influence of sporadic anovulation on hormone levels in ovulatory cycles. Hum Reprod 2013;28(6): 1687–94.
55. Wingfield JC, Sapolsky RM. Reproduction and resistance to stress: when and how. J Neuroendocrinol 2003;15(8):711–24.
56. Loucks AB. The response of luteinizing hormone pulsatility to 5 days of low energy availability disappears by 14 years of gynecological age. J Clin Endocrinol Metab 2006;91(8):3158–64.
57. Rogol AD, Weltman A, Weltman JY, et al. Durability of the reproductive axis in eumenorrheic women during 1 yr of endurance training. J Appl Physiol (1985) 1992;72(4):1571–80.
58. Loucks AB, Cameron JL, De Souza MJ. Subject assignment may have biased exercise results. J Appl Physiol (1985) 1993;74(4):2045–7.
59. Williams NI, Reed JL, Leidy HJ, et al. Estrogen and progesterone exposure is reduced in response to energy deficiency in women aged 25-40 years. Hum Reprod 2010;25(9):2328–39.
60. Caronia LM, Martin C, Welt CK, et al. A genetic basis for functional hypothalamic amenorrhea. N Engl J Med 2011;364(3):215–25.
61. Schwanzelfukuda M, Bick D, Pfaff DW. Luteinizing-hormone-releasing hormone (Lhrh)-expressing cells do not migrate normally in an inherited hypogonadal (Kallmann) syndrome. Mol Brain Res 1989;6(4):311–26.
62. Matsumoto S, Yamazaki C, Masumoto KH, et al. Abnormal development of the olfactory bulb and reproductive system in mice lacking prokineticin receptor PKR2. Proc Natl Acad Sci U S A 2006;103(11):4140–5.
63. Kim SH, Hu Y, Cadman S, et al. Diversity in fibroblast growth factor receptor 1 regulation: learning from the investigation of Kallmann syndrome. J Neuroendocrinol 2008;20(2):141–63.
64. Cheng CK, Leung PCK. Molecular biology of gonadotropin-releasing hormone (GnRH)-I, GnRH-1I, and their receptors in humans. Endocr Rev 2005;26(2): 283–306.
65. Berga SL. Stress and ovarian function. Am J Sports Med 1996;24(6 Suppl): S36–7.
66. Cameron JL. Stress and behaviorally induced reproductive dysfunction in primates. Semin Reprod Endocrinol 1997;15(1):37–45.
67. Ferin M. Stress and the gonadal axis in the female rhesus monkey: interface between the immune and neuroendocrine systems. Hum Reprod 1993;8(Suppl 2): 147–50.
68. Ferin M. Clinical review 105: stress and the reproductive cycle. J Clin Endocrinol Metab 1999;84(6):1768–74.
69. Shively CA, Day SM. Social inequalities in health in nonhuman primates. Neurobiol Stress 2015;1:156–63.
70. Schliep KC, Mumford SL, Vladutiu CJ, et al. Perceived stress, reproductive hormones, and ovulatory function: a prospective cohort study. Epidemiology 2015; 26(2):177–84.
71. Xiao E, Xia-Zhang L, Barth A, et al. Stress and the menstrual cycle: relevance of cycle quality in the short- and long-term response to a 5-day endotoxin challenge during the follicular phase in the rhesus monkey. J Clin Endocrinol Metab 1998;83(7):2454–60.
72. Bethea CL, Centeno ML, Cameron JL. Neurobiology of stress-induced reproductive dysfunction in female macaques. Mol Neurobiol 2008;38(3):199–230.

73. Sanders KA, Bruce NW. A prospective study of psychosocial stress and fertility in women. Hum Reprod 1997;12(10):2324–9.

74. Williams NI, Berga SL, Cameron JL. Synergism between psychosocial and metabolic stressors: impact on reproductive function in cynomolgus monkeys. Am J Physiol Endocrinol Metab 2007;293(1):E270–6.

75. Bethea CL, Streicher JM, Mirkes SJ, et al. Serotonin-related gene expression in female monkeys with individual sensitivity to stress. Neuroscience 2005;132(1):151–66.

76. Bethea CL, Kim A, Reddy AP, et al. Hypothalamic KISS1 expression, gonadotrophin-releasing hormone and neurotransmitter innervation vary with stress and sensitivity in macaques. J Neuroendocrinol 2014;26(5):267–81.

77. Giles DE, Berga SL. Cognitive and psychiatric correlates of functional hypothalamic amenorrhea: a controlled comparison. Fertil Steril 1993;60(3):486–92.

78. Berga SL, Loucks TL. The diagnosis and treatment of stress-induced anovulation. Minerva Ginecol 2005;57(1):45–54.

79. Berga SL, Marcus MD, Loucks TL, et al. Recovery of ovarian activity in women with functional hypothalamic amenorrhea who were treated with cognitive behavior therapy. Fertil Steril 2003;80(4):976–81.

80. Michopoulos V, Mancini F, Loucks TL, et al. Neuroendocrine recovery initiated by cognitive behavioral therapy in women with functional hypothalamic amenorrhea: a randomized, controlled trial. Fertil Steril 2013;99(7):2084–91.e1.

81. Kalantaridou SN, Zoumakis E, Makrigiannakis A, et al. Corticotropin-releasing hormone, stress and human reproduction: an update. J Reprod Immunol 2010;85(1):33–9.

82. Herod SM, Dettmer AM, Novak MA, et al. Sensitivity to stress-induced reproductive dysfunction is associated with a selective but not a generalized increase in activity of the adrenal axis. Am J Physiol Endocrinol Metab 2011;300(1):E28–36.

83. Xiao E, Xia-Zhang L, Vulliemoz N, et al. Astressin B, a corticotropin-releasing hormone receptor antagonist, accelerates the return to normal luteal function after an inflammatory-like stress challenge in the rhesus monkey. Endocrinology 2007;148(2):841–8.

84. Castellano JM, Bentsen AH, Mikkelsen JD, et al. Kisspeptins: bridging energy homeostasis and reproduction. Brain Res 2010;1364:129–38.

85. Loucks AB, Redman LM. The effect of stress on menstrual function. Trends Endocrinol Metab 2004;15(10):466–71.

86. Berga SL. Stress and reproduction: a tale of false dichotomy? Endocrinology 2008;149(3):867–8.

87. Pauli SA, Berga SL. Athletic amenorrhea: energy deficit or psychogenic challenge? Ann N Y Acad Sci 2010;1205:33–8.

88. De Souza MJ, Lee DK, VanHeest JL, et al. Severity of energy-related menstrual disturbances increases in proportion to indices of energy conservation in exercising women. Fertil Steril 2007;88(4):971–5.

89. Loucks AB, Laughlin GA, Mortola JF, et al. Hypothalamic-pituitary-thyroidal function in eumenorrheic and amenorrheic athletes. J Clin Endocrinol Metab 1992;75(2):514–8.

90. Laughlin GA, Yen SS. Nutritional and endocrine-metabolic aberrations in amenorrheic athletes. J Clin Endocrinol Metab 1996;81(12):4301–9.

91. Myerson M, Gutin B, Warren MP, et al. Resting metabolic rate and energy balance in amenorrheic and eumenorrheic runners. Med Sci Sports Exerc 1991;23(1):15–22.

92. Rickenlund A, Eriksson MJ, Schenck-Gustafsson K, et al. Amenorrhea in female athletes is associated with endothelial dysfunction and unfavorable lipid profile. J Clin Endocrinol Metab 2005;90(3):1354–9.

93. Zeni Hoch A, Dempsey RL, Carrera GF, et al. Is there an association between athletic amenorrhea and endothelial cell dysfunction? Med Sci Sports Exerc 2003;35(3):377–83.

94. O'Donnell E, Goodman JM, Harvey PJ. Clinical review: cardiovascular consequences of ovarian disruption: a focus on functional hypothalamic amenorrhea in physically active women. J Clin Endocrinol Metab 2011;96(12):3638–48.

95. De Souza MJ, Williams NI. Physiological aspects and clinical sequelae of energy deficiency and hypoestrogenism in exercising women. Hum Reprod Update 2004;10(5):433–48.

96. Barrack MT, Gibbs JC, De Souza MJ, et al. Higher incidence of bone stress injuries with increasing female athlete triad-related risk factors: a prospective multisite study of exercising girls and women. Am J Sports Med 2014;42(4): 949–58.

97. Mountjoy M, Sundgot-Borgen J, Burke L, et al. The IOC consensus statement: beyond the female athlete triad–relative energy deficiency in sport (RED-S). Br J Sports Med 2014;48(7):491–7.

98. Marcason W. Female athlete triad or relative energy deficiency in sports (RED-S): is there a difference? J Acad Nutr Diet 2016;116(4):744.

99. Valliant MW. The female athlete triad and relative energy deficiency in sport: knowledge of both can improve the health of female athletes. Strength Conditioning J 2016;38(2):35–8.

100. Tenforde AS, Barrack MT, Nattiv A, et al. Parallels with the female athlete triad in male athletes. Sports Med 2016;46(2):171–82.

101. Cano Sokoloff N, Misra M, Ackerman KE. Exercise, training, and the hypothalamic-pituitary-gonadal axis in men and women. Front Horm Res 2016;47:27–43.

102. Meeusen R, Duclos M, Foster C, et al. Prevention, diagnosis, and treatment of the overtraining syndrome: joint consensus statement of the European College of Sport Science and the American College of Sports Medicine. Med Sci Sports Exerc 2013;45(1):186–205.

103. Hackney AC. Effects of endurance exercise on the reproductive system of men: the "exercise-hypogonadal male condition". J Endocrinol Invest 2008;31(10): 932–8.

104. Ackerman KE, Skrinar GS, Medvedova E, et al. Estradiol levels predict bone mineral density in male collegiate athletes: a pilot study. Clin Endocrinol (Oxf) 2012;76(3):339–45.

105. Smink FR, van Hoeken D, Hoek HW. Epidemiology of eating disorders: incidence, prevalence and mortality rates. Curr Psychiatry Rep 2012;14(4):406–14.

106. Martinsen M, Sundgot-Borgen J. Higher prevalence of eating disorders among adolescent elite athletes than controls. Med Sci Sports Exerc 2013;45(6): 1188–97.

107. Bonci CM, Bonci LJ, Granger LR, et al. National Athletic Trainers' Association position statement: preventing, detecting, and managing disordered eating in athletes. J Athl Train 2008;43(1):80–108.

108. Garner D, Olmsted MP, Polivy J. The eating disorder inventory: a measure of cognitive-behavioral dimensions of anorexia nervosa and bulimia. Anorexia nervosa: recent developments in research. New York: Alan R. Linse, Inc; 1983. p. 173–84.

109. Stunkard AJ, Messick S. The three-factor eating questionnaire to measure dietary restraint, disinhibition and hunger. J Psychosom Res 1985;29(1):71–83.

110. Cooper Z, Fairburn C. The eating disorder examination: a semi-structured interview for the assessment of the specific psychopathology of eating disorders. Int J Eat Disord 1987;6(1):1–8.

111. Martinsen M, Holme I, Pensgaard AM, et al. The development of the brief eating disorder in athletes questionnaire. Med Sci Sports Exerc 2014;46(8):1666–75.

112. Melin A, Tornberg AB, Skouby S, et al. The LEAF questionnaire: a screening tool for the identification of female athletes at risk for the female athlete triad. Br J Sports Med 2014;48(7):540–5.

113. Bratland-Sanda S, Sundgot-Borgen J. Eating disorders in athletes: overview of prevalence, risk factors and recommendations for prevention and treatment. Eur J Sport Sci 2013;13(5):499–508.

114. Martinsen M, Sherman RT, Thompson RA, et al. Coaches' knowledge and management of eating disorders: a randomized controlled trial. Med Sci Sports Exerc 2015;47(5):1070–8.

115. Martinsen M, Bahr R, Borresen R, et al. Preventing eating disorders among young elite athletes: a randomized controlled trial. Med Sci Sports Exerc 2014;46(3):435–47.

116. Tenforde AS, Carlson JL, Chang A, et al. Association of the female athlete triad risk assessment stratification to the development of bone stress injuries in collegiate athletes. Am J Sports Med 2017;45(2):302–10.

117. Kraus EA, Kim B, Nattiv A, et al. Higher cumulative risk assessment scores are associated with delayed return to play in division I collegiate distance runners. PM R 2016;8(9S):S212–3.

Osteopenia and Osteoporosis in Female Athletes

John M. MacKnight, MD

KEYWORDS

- Osteopenia • Osteoporosis • Low bone density • Athlete • Sports medicine

KEY POINTS

- Low bone mass manifest as osteopenia or osteoporosis is common in the general population and especially common in female athletes.
- Exercise is an important stimulus to bone formation, but when done to excess may impact negatively on bone health as both a young and older woman.
- Attention to optimizing maximal bone mass development as an adolescent and young adult is crucial to establishing lifelong bone health for women.
- Bone health is positively influenced by a number of lifestyle measures; it should be every care provider's goal to optimize these important factors for women throughout their lives.

Disorders of bone density are common in the general population and especially prevalent among athletic women.[1] The severity of bone loss is variable and ranges from milder degrees of bone loss, termed osteopenia, to more profound degrees of loss resulting in frank osteoporosis. More than half of US adults older than 50 years have low bone mass at the femoral neck or lumbar spine, and nearly 10% meet the diagnostic criteria for osteoporosis at one or both sites.[2] In female athletes, there is a higher incidence of osteoporosis due to a decreased rate of bone accretion in youth, which in turn results in a lower peak bone mass, especially in those with delayed menarche.[3] Low bone mass poses a particular challenge for athletes because it not only predisposes to stress-related bone injuries but also sets the stage for increased risk of osteoporosis and insufficiency fractures with aging.

Disclosure Statement: The author has no relationship with a commercial company that has a direct financial interest in subject matter or materials discussed in this article or with a company making a competing product.
Internal Medicine, University of Virginia Health System, University Physicians-Charlottesville, 415 Ray C. Hunt Drive, Suite 2100, Charlottesville, VA 22908, USA
E-mail address: jm9m@virginia.edu

This article reviews the pathophysiology of bone thinning in both premenopausal and postmenopausal women, the impact of exercise on these processes, and the treatment options presently available. It should be every provider's goal to proactively identify at-risk individuals to prevent major bone metabolic issues before they arise. For women who already demonstrate bone thinning, the collective goal must be to correct present deficiencies, modify future osteoporosis risk, and preserve the desired level of activity.

NORMAL BONE METABOLISM

The adult human skeleton is composed of 2 types of bone. Cortical bone accounts for roughly 80% of overall bone mass and is dense, solid, and surrounds the bone marrow space. Trabecular or cancellous bone is a honeycomblike network of trabecular plates and rods throughout the bone marrow compartment[4] that makes up the remaining 20%. Bone is a dynamic tissue that is involved in a constant remodeling process of formation and resorption.[5–7] Bone remodeling is initiated at the cellular level by osteoclasts that contain enzymes that dissolve the bone surface and drive the resorption process. To compensate for bone breakdown, osteoblasts initiate bone formation by secreting osteoid, the bone matrix protein, which then mineralizes to complete the bone formation process.[5,8] The most crucial time in this process for maximum gains in peak bone mass and the development of long-term bone density is in adolescence and early adulthood. Healthy girls experience a peak period of bone mass accrual typically between ages 11 and 14 years,[9] with nearly 90% of peak bone mass attained by the age of 18.[10] Increases in growth hormone, insulinlike growth factor 1, and estrogen that occur between Tanner stages 2 and 4 coincide with these maximal rates of bone mineral gain. Despite strong genetic determinants of individual bone mineral density (BMD), it is during this critical time that a number of intrinsic or extrinsic factors may play a negative role in the achievement of maximal bone mass as well. These factors will be addressed later in this article.

After maximum bone mass is achieved by approximately age 35 years, the remodeling process becomes uncoupled and bone density begins a slow and steady decline that may eventually lead to osteopenia or osteoporosis.[11–15] The preservation of bone density and the ability to perform athletically over time are a direct result of optimizing bone deposition early in life and minimizing this inevitable decline in bone density, especially after menopause. It is estimated based on present data that achieving a 10% higher peak bone mass in young adulthood may delay the development of osteoporosis by approximately 13 years, and ultimately reduce the lifetime risk of fracture by 50%.[16]

IMPACT OF SPORT AND EXERCISE ON BONE HEALTH

Sedentarism is associated with the risk of developing osteoporosis. Physical activity is the only lifestyle measure that increases bone mass and strength while also reducing the risk of falls later in life. Bone responds to mechanotransduction, a process by which bone recognizes mechanical loading through mechanoreceptors in osteocytes. Osteogenic, bone-forming, stresses are variable, dynamic, and progressive; static exercise loading does not cause osteogenesis.[17] In children and adolescents, mechanical loading of bone through physical activity is essential for maximal bone density acquisition. The benefits seen in childhood and adolescence continue into adulthood and are important for the maintenance of bone density with aging.[18–21] As such, the recommendation of exercise for the prevention of osteoporosis later in life should begin in childhood and continue through life. Although relatively less protective, even exercise training begun after menopause may help to prevent future fractures.[22]

The greatest value from exercise is derived from discrete bouts of activity with recovery periods in between, and is most beneficial during the time of skeletal growth. As bone will adapt to repeated similar patterns of loading, it is important to incorporate activities with multidirectional loading to continue to stimulate an adaptive skeletal response.[23] The precise amount of exercise that is optimal has yet to be determined, but it is well understood that the effects of exercise on bone are modality-dependent, dose-dependent and intensity-dependent.[24] Exercise goals for maximal benefit include the following[25]:

- Dynamic, not static exercise
- Adequate strain intensity
- Discrete, intermittent bouts
- Variable loading patterns
- Optimal nutrition with adequate intake of calcium and vitamin D

The American College of Sports Medicine recommends weight-bearing endurance and plyometric exercise 3 to 5 times per week, and resistance exercise of moderate to high loading 2 to 3 times per week for a total of 30 to 60 minutes per day.[26] Modifications may be necessary to ensure safety in the elderly; nonetheless, a regular pattern of exercise should be continued to improve balance and prevent falls.

Strength and power-trained athletes as well as athletes with habitually heavy training levels typically demonstrate the highest bone mineral densities. Cross-sectional studies also consistently demonstrate that athletes engaged in high-impact weight-bearing sports with rapid rates of loading, such as gymnastics, volleyball, basketball, ballet dancing, football, power lifting, tennis/squash, and figure skating have superior bone mass at loaded skeletal sites compared with nonathletes or athletes in lower-impact sports.[27-33]

Programs that incorporate moderate-to-high weight-bearing impact loads (>2 times body weight), that are progressive, novel, and multidirectional may be osteogenic for both premenopausal women and older adults.[34,35] Randomized controlled trials and meta-analyses also have shown that impact exercise training, such as hopping and jumping, and/or progressive resistance training enhance the bone health of children and adolescents,[36] as well as premenopausal,[37] and postmenopausal women.[38] Such activities have the most impact on femoral neck BMD, whereas a combination exercise program is most effective for BMD at the spine.[39] Weight-bearing activity during adolescence and early adulthood is an important predictor of peak bone mass; young women participating regularly in sports at school demonstrated higher bone mass than those who did not.[40] It is important to remember, however, that excessive exercise in premenopausal women may lead to energy deficiency, weight loss, and amenorrhea, which may contribute to bone loss and osteoporosis rather than preventing it (see Nancy I. Williams and colleagues' article, "Female Athlete Triad: Future Directions for Energy Availability and Eating Disorder Research and Practice," in this issue).

PATHOPHYSIOLOGY OF BONE LOSS

Osteopenia and osteoporosis are characterized by decreased bone mass, disruption of the bony microarchitecture with loss of trabeculae, and skeletal fragility, which results in diminished bone strength and an increased risk of fracture. Both conditions arise from inadequate bone development/deposition, excessive bone breakdown, or a combination of the two. Decreased bone mass in athletes is a function of the age of onset of physical training; the duration, volume, and intensity of training; and the physical demands of sport.[41] Several intrinsic and extrinsic factors may also contribute to abnormal bone density (**Box 1**), but most affected women demonstrate relative estrogen deficiency in premenopause or frank and profound estrogen deficiency in postmenopause. Estrogen plays a central role in skeletal homeostasis and BMD through its impact on both osteoblasts and osteoclasts, inhibition of bone

---

Box 1
Secondary causes of osteoporosis

Endocrine

Adrenal insufficiency

Cushing syndrome

Eating disorders

Endometriosis

Hyperparathyroidism

Hyperprolactinemia

Hyperthyroidism

Hypogonadism

Diabetes mellitus

Gastrointestinal/Nutrition

Inflammatory bowel disease

Vitamin D and/or calcium deficiency

Anorexia nervosa

Celiac disease

Malabsorption syndromes

Pancreatic insufficiency

Marrow disorders

Hemochromatosis

Leukemia

Lymphoma

Mastocytosis

Multiple myeloma

Pernicious anemia

Miscellaneous causes

Ankylosing spondylitis

Idiopathic hypercalciuria

Idiopathic scoliosis

Multiple sclerosis

Rheumatoid arthritis

From Fitzpatrick LA. Secondary causes of osteoporosis. Mayo Clin Proc 2002;77:453.

turnover, and favorable effects on the balance between bone deposition and break-down.[42] Estrogen also exerts indirect effects on other bone-modifying hormones, including calcitonin, parathyroid hormone (PTH), cytokines, and growth factors.[43,44] Because exercise has profound effects on the postexercise pulsatile behavior of luteinizing hormone, follicle-stimulating hormone, and estradiol, intensive aerobic exercise may impact negatively on bone density through the low estrogen levels generated by hypothalamic-pituitary-gonadal axis dysfunction.[42,45] Some premenopausal women with low BMD may suffer from a genetically determined low peak bone mass with no other obvious cause. Similarly, premenopausal women with bone fragility but no known secondary causes are diagnosed with idiopathic osteoporosis. Proposed mechanisms include osteoblast dysfunction, subclinical estrogen deficiency, increased bone turnover, and abnormalities in growth hormone/insulinlike growth factor 1.[46–50]

Long-standing increases in cortisol affect calcium and bone metabolism, increase bone resorption, decrease bone formation, and contribute to osteopenia and osteoporosis. Elevated cortisol levels result from intense exercise and may be seen in athletes who are overtrained. Cortisol is also increased in amenorrheic athletes. Leptin, the adipocyte-secreted protein product of the obesity gene, decreases in response to starvation, which then results in a decrease in estradiol levels and amenorrhea.[51] Leptin levels in athletic women are also further decreased by low amounts of fat storage.[52] These metabolic changes are theorized to contribute to low BMD in excessively thin, athletic women.

DIAGNOSIS

Because osteopenia and osteoporosis pose a significant risk for the health and athleticism of active women, it is essential that a diagnosis be made as early in the bone loss process as possible. Screening processes for detection of low BMD are not uniform, but should be applied to at-risk populations whenever feasible; screening for low BMD should not be routinely performed in asymptomatic premenopausal women. The evaluation for low bone mass or fracture risk in women should begin with a detailed history, physical examination, and biochemical assessment, including complete blood count profile, complete chemistry profile including alkaline phosphatase, 25-hydroxy-vitamin D, serum calcium, phosphorus, and thyroid stimulating hormone. Based on those results, additional testing to explore other potential underlying conditions may be needed to explore gonadotropic hormones, iron, parathyroid, 24-hour urinary calcium and creatinine, and autoimmune status. A sizable proportion of premenopausal women with osteoporosis have an identifiable secondary cause, and[47,53] appropriate identification of the underlying condition will aid in guiding appropriate management.

Dual-Energy X-Ray Absorptiometry Scanning

Measurement of BMD is generally accomplished via dual-energy x-ray absorptiometry (DXA) scanning. Without fragility fracture, low BMD determination by DXA is the standard testing modality to diagnose osteoporosis.[54,55] For women who may have achieved a lower than desirable bone mass due to external factors during the critical developmental time in adolescence, the use of serial BMD assessments by DXA may be necessary. Those with ongoing bone loss will be expected to show a progressive decline in BMD over time, whereas those with past bone metabolism issues would be expected to demonstrate stable BMD with serial evaluations. In circumstances in which only a single BMD value is available, elevations of serum or urinary markers of bone turnover (eg, N-telopeptide) suggest that active bone breakdown is occurring.

However, the range of normal values for premenopausal women is broad and may make interpretation challenging.[50] Adolescents and young adults are expected to have active bone modeling and remodeling with expected increases in bone turnover markers. Recent fractures also would be expected to elevate bone turnover markers.

T-Score

The T-score was established by the World Health Organization (WHO) to compare the SD difference between patient BMD as determined by DXA versus a young adult reference group.[55]

- T-score within 1 SD of the reference group: Normal
- T-score −1.0 to −2.5: Osteopenia
- T-score ≤−2.5: Osteoporosis

The degree of decline in BMD as determined by T-score correlates with relative fracture risk; consequently, those with a T-score ≤−2.5 have the highest fracture risk. WHO thresholds were established based on relative fracture risk in postmenopausal white women. As such, these criteria may not be readily applicable to other genetic groups.

Z-Score

The Z-score compares patient BMD with a group of age-matched peers. In children younger than 20, the Z-score rather than the T-score should be used, as direct comparisons cannot be made between a group that has not yet reached peak bone mass and an adult group that has. At this time, data to allow for the calculation of Z-scores in children are limited.[56] In premenopausal women, the International Society for Clinical Densitometry advises the use of BMD Z-scores at the lumbar spine, total hip, femoral neck, and distal radius rather than using the T-score noted previously. A Z-score less than −2.0 is considered "below the expected BMD for age" and should prompt a search for secondary causes of bone loss.[57] BMD measurements alone should not be used to define osteoporosis in premenopausal women,[54] but rather low BMD for age (Z-score ≤−2.0) coupled with risk factors for fracture or established secondary causes of osteoporosis.[58]

Fracture Risk Assessment Tool

The Fracture Risk Assessment Tool (FRAX)[59] was developed to calculate relative fracture probability using femoral neck BMD data as determined by DXA. FRAX is a computer-based calculator that estimates the 10-year probability of hip fracture and major osteoporotic fracture (hip, spine, proximal humerus, or forearm) for untreated patients between the ages of 40 and 90 years. FRAX cannot be used in the premenopausal population.

Newer imaging strategies include high-resolution peripheral quantitative computed tomography, which can better distinguish healthy microarchitecture of bone from suboptimal bone using 3-dimensional information to estimate bone geometry.[60] An additional tool to assess bone integrity is the trabecular bone score, a gray-level textural measurement that indirectly evaluates bone microarchitecture.[61] Both are in their early stages of use.

FRACTURES

Osteoporosis is generally a "silent" process with no clinical manifestations until the athlete suffers a fracture. Trabecular bone in vertebral bodies, the neck of the femur, and the distal radius are most frequently affected by osteoporosis. Vertebral fractures are the most common manifestation of osteoporosis, although most patients with evidence of vertebral fracture are asymptomatic and have the diagnosis made incidentally by imaging obtained for other reasons. Hip fracture risk in osteoporotic women rises dramatically as patients age, with up to 15% of women having suffered such an injury by age 80.[62] Distal radius fractures (Colles fractures) are also seen in this group, although the relative risk is highest in early perimenopause. The clinical significance of low bone mass in premenopausal women is unknown. Presently the available data in premenopausal women with low BMD and no known secondary causes have failed to show a predictable risk of insufficiency fracture.[46,63,64]

A history of fragility fracture is a prominent risk factor for a subsequent fracture.[65,66] According to the Study of Osteoporotic Fractures, women with a history of premenopausal fracture were 35% more likely to fracture again during their postmenopausal years.[67] Similarly, in a large meta-analysis involving more than 44,000 women, previous fracture was associated with an almost twofold increased risk of any fracture (relative risk [RR] 1.86) relative to those without a prior fracture.[68]

It is estimated that more than 50% of women who suffer a low-trauma fragility fracture are actually osteopenic rather than osteoporotic.[69] As such, it is postulated that other skeletal factors aside from low BMD, such as cross-sectional area, macroarchitecture and micro-architecture, and intrinsic properties, such as matrix mineralization, collagen characteristics, and degree of porosity, also exert important effects on bone strength and relative risk for fracture. External factors, such as muscular strength and balance are also important determinants of risk.[70]

Stress injuries result from a disturbance in the balance between osteoblastic bone formation and osteoclastic bone resorption in the face of repeated mechanical loading of the bone. If bone is unable to withstand the repetitive mechanical stresses of sport, fracture can occur. Cancellous bone stress fractures occur more often in patients with osteopenia, as opposed to cortical stress fractures.[71,72] More severe stress fractures have been found to correlate with lower BMD, and those stress fractures considered to be of highest risk (sacrum, pelvis, femoral neck) are often associated with the bone loss risk factors seen in the Female Athlete Triad.[72] Although stress fracture risk in athletes and active individuals may be associated with low BMD, the data are variable and many athletes who suffer stress fractures actually have normal BMD.[73–75] Stress injuries of bone are common in athletes with a prevalence of 0.7% to 21.0%,[76] highest in track and field athletes. Runners with oligomenorrhea have been found to be 6 times more likely to sustain a stress injury as a result of their suboptimal hormonal status.[77]

TREATMENT
Nonpharmacologic Treatment

Calcium, vitamin D, and maximal lifestyle management with emphasis on weight-bearing exercise are recommended as the fundamental interventions for all women with low BMD.

Lifestyle management

Lifestyle management should be recommended for all women with low BMD. Important lifestyle measures include regular weight-bearing exercise, counseling on fall prevention, achievement or maintenance of normal body weight, minimizing or eliminating the use of extreme dieting, smoking cessation, and moderate alcohol consumption. As their medical status will allow, women should also try to avoid the use of medications known to contribute to bone loss with particular attention to aluminum-containing antacids, antiepileptics, glucocorticoids, a number of hormonal therapies, immunosuppressives, proton pump inhibitors, and selective serotonin uptake inhibitors.

Vitamin D

Vitamin D is essential for bone growth, density, and remodeling and plays a central role in skeletal bone mineralization and calcium metabolism.[78] Although there is some variation among recommendations for vitamin D intake, it is generally accepted that premenopausal women should consume 600 IU of vitamin D daily, whereas postmenopausal women should consume 800 to 1000 IU daily.[54] As it can be difficult to reach this goal with diet alone, most postmenopausal women also should use vitamin D supplementation. Although accepted as beneficial for bone density, a debate still exists over the benefit of vitamin D and calcium in reducing the risk of fractures.[79–81]

Calcium

The goal for optimal calcium intake in premenopausal women is 1000 mg per day. Postmenopausal women should consume 1200 mg daily.[54] Women who are meeting this intake through diet alone do not need to supplement with additional calcium. Those who are not should use elemental calcium supplements such that the total daily calcium intake from food and supplementation is approximately 1200 mg per day.[82] Some concern has been raised regarding increased cardiovascular risk associated with calcium supplementation; this remains controversial.

Exercise

The beneficial effects of exercise on bone density in women with low BMD are small with high-intensity exercise no more beneficial than low-intensity activities. Because continuation of a regular pattern of exercise is important to maintain whatever gains are made, efforts should be made to ensure that such activities can be done on a regular basis and are enjoyable.[83] Exercise recommendations should follow the guidelines previously outlined. It is also important to remember that excessive exercise in premenopausal women may lead to weight loss and estrogen deficiency from hypothalamic amenorrhea, which will in turn exacerbate low bone density rather than correct it.

Experts have suggested that the one absolute contraindication for osteoporotic athletes and active individuals is trunk flexion exercise, which may predispose to lumbar vertebral insufficiency fracture.[84] Additional research over 10 years of study showed that extension exercises appear to be safe, and they observed a lower number of fractures in women who trained with extension exercise versus no exercise.[85] It is also prudent to advise osteoporotic patients to avoid exercises such as push-ups, curl-ups, and vertical jump and to engage in low-impact weight-bearing activities and resistance training.

Pharmacologic Treatment

Although multiple pharmacologic therapies are available for the treatment of postmenopausal women, there are few data to support the use of these therapies in premenopausal women except in cases of osteoporotic fracture, evidence of active bone loss, and/or known secondary causes of osteoporosis. In women with a diagnosed secondary cause of osteoporosis (see **Box 1**), the treatment of choice is targeted toward the underlying condition. In consideration of pharmacologic management of postmenopausal low BMD, the National Osteoporosis Foundation[54] recommends the following guidelines:

- Pharmacologic treatment for postmenopausal women with a history of fragility fracture or with osteoporosis based on BMD measurement (T-score ≤ -2.5).
- Pharmacologic treatment of high-risk postmenopausal women with T-scores between -1.0 and -2.5 who have a high-risk FRAX score indicating a 10-year probability of hip fracture of $\geq 3\%$ or of combined major osteoporotic fracture of $\geq 20\%$.

Treatment cutoffs based on absolute fracture risk, as opposed to BMD measures, have not been assessed in clinical trials. Treatment approaches always should be individualized, but it appears clear that those at highest risk for fracture are likely to benefit the most from aggressive drug therapy.

Bisphosphonates
This powerful class of therapies inhibits osteoclastic resorption of bone by attaching to hydroxyapatite binding sites on bony surfaces and may have a beneficial effect on osteoblast function as well.

In premenopausal women, there are few high-quality safety or efficacy data regarding bisphosphonate use. The decision to use such therapies will involve an individualized risk:benefit assessment based on multiple clinical factors. In premenopausal women, alendronate and risedronate carry Food and Drug Administration approval only for use in those receiving glucocorticoid therapy but not for low BMD without secondary cause. Significant potential long-term risks include atypical femoral fractures and osteonecrosis of the jaw.[86,87] The long half-life of bisphosphonates in bone make their long-term potential side effects in women of reproductive age likely more problematic than their relative efficacy. These therapies are category C for safety in pregnancy.

For postmenopausal women with osteoporosis, oral bisphosphonates should be considered first-line therapy for most based on efficacy, cost, and long-term proven safety. Multiple studies have proven them effective for both the prevention and treatment of osteoporosis by increasing bone mass and reduced incidence of fractures. Alendronate and risedronate have proven value for decreasing the rate of vertebral and hip fracture. Caution must be used in treating patients with esophageal disorders and chronic kidney disease.

Alternatives to oral bisphosphonates
Intravenous bisphosphonates Zoledronic acid and ibandronate should be considered for women with intolerance to oral bisphosphonates or in those with underlying esophageal disorders.

Denosumab This humanized monoclonal antibody against RANKL (receptor activator of nuclear factor kappa-B ligand) is administered intravenously. Denosumab reduces osteoclastogenesis, improves BMD, and reduces the incidence of new vertebral, hip, and nonvertebral fractures in postmenopausal women. Denosumab should not be considered first-line therapy for most with osteoporosis, and is approved only for use in postmenopausal women at high risk for fracture. It is category X for pregnancy.

Teriparatide A recombinant form of PTH, teriparatide, is an anabolic therapy with no antiresorptive effects. It has been shown in several clinical trials to prevent bone loss in a variety of patients with low BMD. Premenopausal women on hormonal therapy for endometriosis, taking glucocorticoids, or with idiopathic osteoporosis[88] have been shown to improve bone density on PTH therapy. In women with severe osteoporosis (T ≤ -3.5 or T ≤ -2.5 plus fragility fracture), teriparatide should be considered initial therapy. Treatment is limited to 24 months and is generally then followed by use of an oral bisphosphonate, as noted previously. Teriparatide has been associated with an increased risk for osteosarcoma, especially in girls who are still growing. As such, use should be avoided in those with open physes or with delayed growth.

Selective estrogen receptor modulator Through their selective estrogen effects, selective estrogen receptor modulators (SERMs) impact bone health by inhibiting bone resorption and reducing the risk of vertebral fracture. Use of the SERM raloxifene is generally limited to osteoporotic women without a fragility fracture history who cannot tolerate any of the bisphosphonate choices or who have an increased risk of invasive breast cancer. They also may lead to worsening bone loss in menstruating women.[89]

Estrogen

Premenopausal women Estrogen replacement may be beneficial in premenopausal women who demonstrate accelerated bone loss in the setting of estrogen deficiency, amenorrhea, or who have a history of fracture. In women with persistent amenorrhea, the intervention of choice is to address the underlying cause. If that is unsuccessful or the individual is unlikely to resume a reasonable menstrual pattern on their own, then estrogen therapy should be considered the treatment of choice. Oral contraceptive therapy in such women significantly reduces bone loss and is safer than in postmenopausal women, but risks must be individualized to each case.

Postmenopausal women Estrogen replacement improves BMD, decreases fracture risk, and improves menopausal symptoms in postmenopausal women. After publication of the Women's Health Initiative and the Million Women Study, use decreased due to concerns about potential risks of breast cancer, cardiac disease, and stroke.[90–93] Because of these concerns and the availability of alternative osteoporosis therapies for use in the postmenopausal population, estrogen replacement is no longer considered a first-line agent for postmenopausal osteoporosis.

Vibration Therapy

Vibration platforms are theorized to produce favorable effects on development of both cancellous and cortical bone.[94] Available data to date, however, have failed to show significant improvements in BMD with vibration platform use relative to sham, walking, or no treatment.[95,96]

Nonrecommended Therapies

Multiple therapies that are either unsafe or have failed to show proven efficacy should be avoided. These include estrogen/progestin combination therapy in postmenopausal women, combination antiresorptive therapy, calcitonin, strontium ranelate, calcitriol, vitamin K, tibolone, folate, vitamin B12, androgens, isoflavones, and fluoride.

Recommendations regarding monitoring of response to therapy vary by organization but is generally accomplished with follow-up DXA scan of the hip and spine after 1 to 2 years. The timing of further follow-up is individualized and should be based on the overall pattern of response to therapy. Routine use of bone turnover markers such as urinary N-telopeptide or serum carboxy-terminal collagen crosslinks is generally not necessary in the follow-up of treated osteoporotic women. At this time, the available data support the notion that positive effects on BMD from therapy correlate with a reduction in fracture risk. Meta-analysis of multiple treatment trials concluded that improvement in spine BMD accounted for a predictable but small part of the reduction in fracture risk.[97] Systematic review of trials published from 2005 to 2014 confirmed the fracture-prevention efficacy of multiple agents compared with placebo.[98] All bisphosphonates, denosumab, raloxifene, and teriparatide reduced the risk of vertebral fractures. Alendronate, risedronate, zoledronic acid, teriparatide, and denosumab reduced the risk of nonvertebral fractures as well.

It is clear that the identification of at-risk women, diagnosis of bone loss, and the initiation of appropriate treatment can have a meaningful impact on health and preservation of the desired level of sport or exercise.

REFERENCES

1. Pentyala S, Mysore P, Pentyala S, et al. Osteoporosis in female athletes. Int J Clin Ther Diagn 2013;1(1):5–11.
2. Looker AC, Borrud LG, Dawson-Hughes B, et al. Osteoporosis or low bone mass at the femur neck or lumbar spine in older adults: United States, 2005-2008. NCHS Data Brief 2012;(93):1–8.
3. Warren MP, Stiehl AL. Exercise and female adolescents: effects on the reproductive and skeletal systems. J Am Med Womens Assoc 1999;54:115–20, 138.
4. Clarke B. Normal bone anatomy and physiology. Clin J Am Soc Nephrol 2008; 3(suppl 3):S131–9.
5. Silverberg SJ, Lindsay R. Postmenopausal osteoporosis. Med Clin North Am 1987;71:41–57.
6. Eriksen EF. Normal and pathological remodeling of human trabecular bone: three dimensional reconstruction of the re-modeling sequence in normals and in metabolic bone disease. Endocr Rev 1987;7:379–408.
7. Frost HM. Treatment of osteoporoses by manipulation of coherent bone cell populations. Clin Orthop Relat Res 1979;143:227–44.
8. Ripamonti U, Ma S, Cunningham NS, et al. Initiation of bone regeneration in adult baboons by osteogenin, a bone morphogenetic protein. Matrix 1992;12:369–80.
9. Theintz G, Buchs B, Rizzoli R, et al. Longitudinal monitoring of bone mass accumulation in healthy adolescents: evidence for a marked reduction after 16 years of age at the levels of lumbar spine and femoral neck in female subjects. J Clin Endocrinol Metab 1992;75:1060.
10. Whiting SJ, Vatanparast H, Baxter-Jones A, et al. Factors that affect bone mineral accrual in the adolescent growth spurt. J Nutr 2004;134:696S–700S.
11. Teitelbaum SL. Bone remodeling and the osteoclast. J Bone Miner Res 1993;2(8 Suppl):S523–5.
12. Ivey JL, Baylink DJ. Postmenopausal osteoporosis: proposed roles of defective coupling and estrogen deficiency. Metab Bone Dis Relat Res 1981;3:3–7.
13. Nordin BE, Need AG, Morris HA, et al. New approaches to the problems of osteoporosis. Clin Orthop Relat Res 1985;200:181–97.
14. Riggs BL, Melton LJ. Involutional osteoporosis. N Engl J Med 1986;314:1676–86.
15. Reddy MS, Morgan SL. Decreased bone mineral density and periodontal management. Periodontol 2000 2013;61:195–218.
16. Hernandez CJ, Beaupre GS, Carter DR. A theoretical analysis of the relative influences of peak BMD, age-related bone loss and menopause on the development of osteoporosis. Osteoporos Int 2003;14(10):843–7.
17. Burr DB, Robling AG, Turner CH. Effects of biomechanical stress on bones in animals. Bone 2002;30:781–6.
18. Johnston CC Jr, Slemenda CW. Peak bone mass, bone loss and risk of fracture. Osteoporos Int 1994;4(suppl 1):43–5.

19. Kanis JA, Johnell O, Oden A, et al. Ten year probabilities of osteoporotic fractures according to BMD and diagnostic thresholds. Osteoporos Int 2001;12:989–95.
20. Nichols DL, Sanborn CF, Essery EV. Bone density and young athletic women. An update. Sports Med 2007;37:1001–14.
21. Nordstrom A, Karlsson C, Nyquist F, et al. Bone loss and fracture risk after reduced physical activity. J Bone Miner Res 2005;20:202–7.
22. Kemmler W, Bebenek M, Kohl M, et al. Exercise and fractures in postmenopausal women. Final results of the controlled Erlangen Fitness and Osteoporosis Prevention Study (EFOPS). Osteoporos Int 2015;26(10):2491–9.
23. Lanyon LE. Using functional loading to influence bone mass and architecture: objectives, mechanisms, and relationship with estrogen of the mechanically adaptive process in bone. Bone 1996;18(1 Suppl):37S–43S.
24. Beck BR, Daly RM, Singh MA, et al. Exercise and Sports Science Australia (ESSA) position statement on exercise prescription for the prevention and management of osteoporosis. J Sci Med Sport 2016;20(5):438–45.
25. Borer KT. Physical activity in the prevention and amelioration of osteoporosis in women: interaction of mechanical, hormonal and dietary factors. Sports Med 2005;35:779–830.
26. Kohrt WM, Bloomfield SA, Little KD, et al. American College of Sports Medicine position stand: physical activity and bone health. Med Sci Sports Exerc 2004;36:1985–96.
27. Snow CM, Williams DP, LaRiviere J, et al. Bone gains and losses follow seasonal training and detraining in gymnasts. Calcif Tissue Int 2001;69(1):7–12.
28. Alfredson H, Nordstrom P, Lorentzon R. Bone mass in female volleyball players: a comparison of total and regional bone mass in female volleyball players and non-active females. Calcif Tissue Int 1997;60(4):338–42.
29. Bagur-Calafat C, Farrerons-Minguella J, Girabent-Farres M, et al. The impact of high level basketball competition, calcium intake, menses, and hormone levels in adolescent bone density: a three-year follow-up. J Sports Med Phys Fitness 2015;55(1–2):58–67.
30. Matthews BL, Bennell KL, McKay HA, et al. Dancing for bone health: a 3-year longitudinal study of bone mineral accrual across puberty in female non-elite dancers and controls. Osteoporos Int 2006;17(7):1043–54.
31. Georgeson EC, Weeks BK, McLellan C, et al. Seasonal change in bone, muscle and fat in professional rugby league players and its relationship to injury: a cohort study. BMJ Open 2012;2(6) [pii:e001400].
32. Tsuzuku S, Ikegami Y, Yabe K. Effects of high-intensity resistance training on bone mineral density in young male powerlifters. Calcif Tissue Int 1998;63(4):283–6.
33. Kontulainen S, Sievanen H, Kannus P, et al. Effect of long-term impact-loading on mass, size, and estimated strength of humerus and radius of female racquet-sports players: a peripheral quantitative computed tomography study between young and old starters and controls. J Bone Miner Res 2003;18(2):352–9.
34. Vainionpaa A, Korpelainen R, Vihriala E, et al. Intensity of exercise is associated with bone density change in premenopausal women. Osteoporos Int 2006;17(3):455–63.
35. Allison SJ, Folland JP, Rennie WJ, et al. High impact exercise increased femoral neck bone mineral density in older men: a randomised unilateral intervention. Bone 2013;53(2):321–8.

36. Behringer M, Gruetzner S, McCourt M, et al. Effects of weight-bearing activities on bone mineral content and density in children and adolescents: a meta-analysis. J Bone Miner Res 2014;29(2):467–78.
37. Kelley GA, Kelley KS, Kohrt WM. Exercise and bone mineral density in premenopausal women: a meta-analysis of randomized controlled trials. Int J Endocrinol 2013;2013:741639.
38. Zhao R, Zhao M, Xu Z. The effects of differing resistance training modes on the preservation of bone mineral density in postmenopausal women: a meta-analysis. Osteoporos Int 2015;26(5):1605–18.
39. Howe TE, Shea B, Dawson LJ, et al. Exercise for preventing and treating osteoporosis in postmenopausal women. Cochrane Database Syst Rev 2011;(7):CD000333.
40. Heinonen A. Physical activity, targeted bone loading and bone mineral density in premenopausal women. In: Kahn K, McKay H, Kannus P, et al, editors. Physical activity and bone health. Champaign (IL): Human Kinetics; 2001. p. 129–42.
41. Osteoporosis in Athletes. Irish Osteoporosis Society. Expert views. Available at: http://www.irishosteoporosis.ie/index.php/expert_views/osteoporosis_in_athletes. Accessed February 16, 2017.
42. Riggs BL, Khosla S, Melton LJ. Sex steroids and the construction and conservation of the adult skeleton. Endocr Rev 2002;23:279–302.
43. Balasch J. Sex steroids and bone: current perspectives. Hum Reprod Update 2003;9:207–22.
44. Liu SL, Lebrun CM. Effect of oral contraceptives and hormone replacement therapy on bone mineral density in premenopausal and perimenopausal women: a systematic review. Br J Sports Med 2006;40:11–24.
45. Women OM. Women. In: MacAuley D, editor. Oxford handbook of sports and exercise medicine. New York: Oxford University Press; 2007. p. 749–72.
46. Cohen A, Dempster DW, Recker RR, et al. Abnormal bone microarchitecture and evidence of osteoblast dysfunction in premenopausal women with idiopathic osteoporosis. J Clin Endocrinol Metab 2011;96:3095.
47. Khosla S, Lufkin EG, Hodgson SF, et al. Epidemiology and clinical features of osteoporosis in young individuals. Bone 1994;15:551.
48. Reed BY, Zerwekh JE, Sakhaee K, et al. Serum IGF 1 is low and correlated with osteoblastic surface in idiopathic osteoporosis. J Bone Miner Res 1995;10:1218.
49. Pepene CE, Seck T, Diel I, et al. Concentration of insulin-like growth factor (IGF)-I in iliac crest bone matrix in premenopausal women with idiopathic osteoporosis. Exp Clin Endocrinol Diabetes 2004;112:38.
50. Rubin MR, Schussheim DH, Kulak CA, et al. Idiopathic osteoporosis in premenopausal women. Osteoporos Int 2005;16:526.
51. De Souza MJ, Williams NI. Beyond hypoestrogenism in amenorrheic athletes: energy deficiency as a contributing factor for bone loss. Curr Sports Med Rep 2005; 4:38–44.
52. Matejek N, Weimann E, Witzel C, et al. Hypoleptinaemia in patients with anorexia nervosa and in elite gymnasts with anorexia athletica. Int J Sports Med 1999;20: 451–6.
53. Khan AA, Syed Z. Bone densitometry in premenopausal women: synthesis and review. J Clin Densitom 2004;7:85.
54. Cosman F, de Beur SJ, LeBoff MS, et al. Clinician's guide to prevention and treatment of osteoporosis. Osteoporos Int 2014;25:2359.

55. World Health Organization. Assessment of fracture risk and its application to screening for postmenopausal osteoporosis. Available at: http://apps.who.int/iris/handle/10665/39142. Accessed March 5, 2017.

56. Kalkwarf HJ, Zemel BS, Gilsanz V, et al. The bone mineral density in childhood study: bone mineral content and density according to age, sex, and race. J Clin Endocrinol Metab 2007;92:2087.

57. Binkley N, Bilezikian JP, Kendler DL, et al. Summary of the International Society for Clinical Densitometry 2005 Position Development Conference. J Bone Miner Res 2007;22:643.

58. 2013 ISCE Official Positions - Adult. Available at: http://www.iscd.org/official-positions/2013-iscd-official-positions-adult/. Accessed March 5, 2017.

59. FRAX. Available at: https://www.shef.ac.uk/FRAX. Accessed March 5, 2017.

60. MacNeil JA, Boyd SK. Accuracy of high-resolution peripheral quantitative computed tomography for measurement of bone quality. Med Eng Phys 2007; 29:1096–105.

61. Bousson V, Bergot C, Sutter B, et al. Scientific Committee of the Groupe de Recherche et d'Information sur les Osteoporoses. Trabecular bone score (TBS): available knowledge, clinical relevance, and future prospects. Osteoporos Int 2012;23:1489–501.

62. Svedbom A, Hernlund E, Ivergård M, et al, EU Review Panel of IOF. Osteoporosis in the European Union: a compendium of country-specific reports. Arch Osteoporos 2013;8:137.

63. Peris P, Monegal A, Martínez MA, et al. Bone mineral density evolution in young premenopausal women with idiopathic osteoporosis. Clin Rheumatol 2007;26:958.

64. Cohen A, Liu XS, Stein EM, et al. Bone microarchitecture and stiffness in premenopausal women with idiopathic osteoporosis. J Clin Endocrinol Metab 2009;94:4351.

65. Lindsay R, Silverman SL, Cooper C, et al. Risk of new vertebral fracture in the year following a fracture. JAMA 2001;285:320.

66. Black DM, Arden NK, Palermo L, et al. Prevalent vertebral deformities predict hip fractures and new vertebral deformities but not wrist fractures. Study of Osteoporotic Fractures Research Group. J Bone Miner Res 1999;14:821.

67. Hosmer WD, Genant HK, Browner WS. Fractures before menopause: a red flag for physicians. Osteoporos Int 2002;13:337.

68. Kanis JA, Johnell O, De Laet C, et al. A meta-analysis of previous fracture and subsequent fracture risk. Bone 2004;35:375.

69. Sanders KM, Nicholson GC, Watts JJ, et al. Half the burden of fragility fractures in the community occur in women without osteoporosis. When is fracture prevention cost-effective? Bone 2006;38(5):694–700.

70. Nguyen T, Sambrook P, Kelly P, et al. Prediction of osteoporotic fractures by postural instability and bone density. BMJ 1993;307(6912):1111–5.

71. Marx RG, Saint-Phard D, Callahan LR, et al. Stress fracture sites related to underlying bone health in athletic females. Clin J Sport Med 2001;11:73–6.

72. Nattiv A, Kennedy G, Barrack MT, et al. Correlation of MRI grading of bone stress injuries with clinical risk factors and return to play: a 5-year prospective study in collegiate track and field athletes. Am J Sports Med 2013;41:1930–41.

73. Gam A, Goldstein L, Karmon Y, et al. Comparison of stress fractures of male and female recruits during basic training in the Israeli anti-aircraft forces. Mil Med 2005;170:710.

74. Shaffer RA, Rauh MJ, Brodine SK, et al. Predictors of stress fracture susceptibility in young female recruits. Am J Sports Med 2006;34:108.

75. Joy EA, Campbell D. Stress fractures in the female athlete. Curr Sports Med Rep 2005;4:323.

76. Bennell KL, Brukner PD. Epidemiology and site specificity of stress fractures. Clin Sports Med 1997;16:179–96.

77. Bennell KL, Malcolm SA, Thomas SA, et al. Risk factors for stress fractures in female track-and-field athletes: a retrospective analysis. Clin J Sport Med 1995;5: 229–35.

78. Ogan D, Pritchett K. Vitamin D and the athlete: risks, recommendations, and benefits. Nutrients 2013;5:1856–68.

79. Bischoff-Ferrari HA, Willett WC, Orav EJ, et al. A pooled analysis of vitamin D dose requirements for fracture prevention. N Engl J Med 2012;367:40–9.

80. Bohon TM, Goolsby MA. The role of vitamin D supplements in women's health. Clin Med Insights Womens Health 2013;6:67–70.

81. Grant AM, Avenell A, Campbell MK, et al. Oral vitamin D3 and calcium for secondary prevention of low-trauma fractures in elderly people (randomized evaluation of calcium or vitamin D, RECORD): a randomised placebo-controlled trial. Lancet 2005;365:1621–8.

82. Eastell R. Treatment of postmenopausal osteoporosis. N Engl J Med 1998;338: 736.

83. Dalsky GP, Stocke KS, Ehsani AA, et al. Weight-bearing exercise training and lumbar bone mineral content in postmenopausal women. Ann Intern Med 1988; 108:824.

84. Chilibeck PD, Vatanparast H, Cornish SM, et al. Evidence-based risk assessment and recommendations for physical activity: arthritis, osteoporosis, and low back pain. Appl Physiol Nutr Metab 2011;36(S1):S49–79.

85. Sinaki M, Mikkelsen BA. Postmenopausal spinal osteoporosis: flexion versus extension exercises. Arch Phys Med Rehabil 1984;65(10):593–6.

86. Khosla S, Burr D, Cauley J, et al. Bisphosphonate-associated osteonecrosis of the jaw: report of a task force of the American Society for Bone and Mineral Research. J Bone Miner Res 2007;22:1479.

87. Shane E, Burr D, Ebeling PR, et al. Atypical subtrochanteric and diaphyseal femoral fractures: report of a task force of the American Society for Bone and Mineral Research. J Bone Miner Res 2010;25:2267.

88. Cohen A, Stein EM, Recker RR, et al. Teriparatide for idiopathic osteoporosis in premenopausal women: a pilot study. J Clin Endocrinol Metab 2013;98:1971.

89. Vehmanen L, Elomaa I, Blomqvist C, et al. Tamoxifen treatment after adjuvant chemotherapy has opposite effects on bone mineral density in premenopausal patients depending on menstrual status. J Clin Oncol 2006;24:675.

90. Beral V, Million Women Study Collaborators. Breast cancer and hormone replacement therapy in the Million Women Study. Lancet 2003;362:419–27.

91. Black DM, Rosen CJ. Clinical practice. Postmenopausal osteoporosis. N Engl J Med 2016;374:254–62.

92. Bowring CE, Francis RM. National Osteoporosis Society's position statement on hormone replacement therapy in the prevention and treatment of osteoporosis. Menopause Int 2011;17:63–5.

93. Rossouw JE, Anderson GL, Prentice RL, et al. Risks and benefits of estrogen plus progestin in healthy postmenopausal women: principal results from the women's health initiative randomized controlled trial. JAMA 2002;288:321–33.

94. Christiansen BA, Silva MJ. The effect of varying magnitudes of whole-body vibration on several skeletal sites in mice. Ann Biomed Eng 2006;34:1149.
95. Slatkovska L, Alibhai SM, Beyene J, et al. Effect of whole-body vibration on BMD: a systematic review and meta-analysis. Osteoporos Int 2010;21:1969.
96. von Stengel S, Kemmler W, Engelke K, et al. Effects of whole body vibration on bone mineral density and falls: results of the randomized controlled ELVIS study with postmenopausal women. Osteoporos Int 2011;22:317.
97. Cummings SR, Karpf DB, Harris F, et al. Improvement in spine bone density and reduction in risk of vertebral fractures during treatment with antiresorptive drugs. Am J Med 2002;112:281.
98. Crandall CJ, Newberry SJ, Diamant A, et al. Comparative effectiveness of pharmacologic treatments to prevent fractures: an updated systematic review. Ann Intern Med 2014;161:711.

Update on Anterior Cruciate Ligament Rupture and Care in the Female Athlete

(●) CrossMark

Jeremy M. Burnham, MD[a,b], Vonda Wright, MD, MS[a,*]

KEYWORDS

- ACL • Anterior cruciate ligament • ACL reconstruction • Anterolateral ligament
- Anterolateral complex • Female athlete • ACL outcomes

KEY POINTS

- Anterior cruciate ligament (ACL) rupture rates in females are on the rise.
- ACL reconstruction must not be a one-size-fits-all approach but must be individualized to restore the native ACL anatomy and address any concomitant injury to secondary stabilizers.
- ACL rehabilitation programs should target hip, core, and trunk neuromuscular control; allow adequate time for graft ligamentization; and address the psychosocial needs of the athlete.
- Return-to-sports assessment requires a multipronged approach; no one test can determine return-to-sports readiness, and a battery of tests is required.
- A team approach involving the surgeon, athletic trainer, therapist, patient, family, and coach is paramount in achieving optimal outcomes after ACL reconstruction.

Despite advances in the surgical care of patients with anterior cruciate ligament (ACL) rupture over the last 30 years, prevention of the initial injury remains elusive, especially in athletes 14 to 19 years old. Beginning with Title IX and female athletic participation increasing 10-fold over the last 40 years, ACL tear rates in female athletes have continued to plague female athletes, with rates estimated at 2 to 8 times those experienced by male athletes.[1] This finding is most true in cutting sports with periods of rapid deceleration, such as soccer, with rates twice as high as men. In basketball, rates of female athlete ACL rupture is 3 to 4 times that of male athletes.[2] The cause of these observations is multifactorial and not clearly defined. In addition, while a

Disclosure: The authors have no conflicts of interest to disclose.
[a] UPMC Center for Sports Medicine, 3200 South Water Street, Pittsburgh, PA 15203, USA;
[b] Sports Medicine at Bone & Joint Clinic, 7301 Hennessy Boulevard, 200, Baton Rouge, LA 70808, USA
* Corresponding author. 8000 Cranberry Springs Drive, Cranberry Township, PA 16066.
E-mail address: wrigvj@upmc.edu

consensus exists as to the efficacy of ACL prevention programs in young female athletes, the optimization of program prescription is still unclear.

THE COST OF ANTERIOR CRUCIATE LIGAMENT RUPTURE

The incidence of primary ACL ruptures varies from 250,000 to 300,000 annually. Female athletes are not only at higher risk of sustaining an initial ACL rupture but also of contralateral ACL tear and reconstruction.[3,4] The Multicenter Orthopaedic Outcomes Network cohort found that females were more likely to need another ACL surgery[5,6] after the index procedure in a 7-year follow-up, with 0.7 ACL injuries per season for female soccer players versus 0.4 for men.[7]

Retear rates are also higher in female athletes younger than 25 years and with smaller primary grafts (less than 8 mm in diameter).[8] Even after successful primary reconstruction, 28% of all female soccer players and 34% of reconstructed players who returned to sport had a second ACL tear.[9] These injuries account for more than $2 billion in annual surgical and rehabilitative care dollars.[10,11]

In addition to the financial cost of ACL rupture and reconstruction, athletes experience extensive personal and social costs of injury and rehabilitation with loss of mobility, pain, social isolation, and alterations in scholastic performance, with 36% failing an examination after return from surgery performed midsemester, compared with 0% with surgery performed during a holiday.[12] In addition, female athletes are less likely to return to sports participation after ACL surgery when compared with boys.[13]

CAUSE OF HIGHER ANTERIOR CRUCIATE LIGAMENT RUPTURE RATES IN FEMALE ATHLETES

The reasons females are significantly more likely to experience ACL rupture are multidimensional and complex. Hagglund and Walden[14] identified age greater than 14 years, family history, and preseason knee pain as key risk factors for future rupture. Fatigue in young soccer players may also compromise athletes' neuromuscular feedback pathways and ability to quickly activate their muscles and respond to physical and visual cues, thus, increasing their injury rates.[15]

ACL injury, however, is not likely due to completely random events but is thought to follow specific repetitive movement patterns that result in more than 70% of all ACL ruptures in female athletes occurring in noncontact situations. The most commonly identified knee position during ACL rupture is an eccentric contraction of the quadriceps (quad) in stiff knee landing, a planted foot with internally rotated hip, valgus knee position in near full extension, and with an upright trunk position.[16–18]

Chappell and colleagues[19] identified quad dominance during landing as a factor resulting in increased ACL loading in landing. Quad dominance is an imbalance in the strength of the knee extensors and flexors as well as recruitment and coordination. This imbalance results in an athlete landing with the knee in nearly full extension and placing high forces across the ACL. Functional training focusing in part on hamstring strength has been shown to help improve dynamic valgus control of the knee and reduce the quad dominance patterns found in women.

In addition, biomechanics contribute to the risk. Excessive subtalar pronation and internal tibial rotation increase ACL strain and increase the detrimental effect of the female athletes' anterior knee laxity. These forces, in conjunction with puberty-related neuromuscular deficits, result in dynamic joint instability during unconscious proprioceptive movements. It is unlikely that a single high-energy movement into this position causes the rupture. It is more likely that repetitive jump-landing in this dropped hip and valgus knee position or with every running step (an average of 1000 steps per mile) creates excessive overload stress to the ACL that simply fatigues with time and ruptures in a noncontact situation.[20]

In a study of 721 female high school athletes, Pappas and colleagues[21] investigated these concepts even further and described 3 biomechanical deficit profiles associated with an increased ACL injury risk in female athletes. Sixty percent of the studied female athletes fit into one of the 3 profiles associated with higher risk of injury. Twenty-four percent demonstrated a combination of high quad and leg dominance deficits. These athletes had increased lower extremity asymmetry and decreased hamstring strength relative to quad strength. The second most common deficit profile, the trunk-leg-ligament group, accounted for 22% of athletes and consisted of athletes with trunk, leg, and ligament deficits. This group reinforced the theory that ACL risk is multifactorial and underscored the difficulty in identifying specific factors associated with injury risk. Finally, 14% of athletes were classified as the ligament-dominance group. These athletes had higher dynamic knee valgus angles and moments, thus, were at greatest risk for noncontact ACL injury. The data obtained by Pappas and colleagues[21] may assist clinicians in designing targeted rehabilitation and prevention programs based on patients' biomechanical profiles.

In addition to the neuromuscular factors exposing female athletes to higher risks of rupture, anatomic studies of structure and mechanical properties of female versus male ACLs find that female ACLs are smaller, have lower tensile linear stiffness with less elongation at failure, and lower energy absorption and load at failure than male ligaments.[22] Renstrom and colleagues[2] reported that female knees have greater tibiofemoral joint laxity and lower joint resistance to translation and rotation as defined as greater than 2 mm side-to-side difference on KT-1000 (MEDmetric Corporation, San Diego, CA).

Bone configuration in female athletes is also thought to contribute to the higher incidence of ACL ruptures in this group. Smaller femoral notch size and greater posterior tibial slope of the lateral knee with resultant increased anterior tibial translation are cited as contributors to suboptimal knee mechanics.[23–25]

Multiple studies have pointed to the role of sex hormones, estrogen, testosterone, and progesterone in the incidence of ACL rupture. Hormone levels of estrogen, testosterone, and progesterone in male and female athletes are not well understood and vary greatly depending on exertion level, nutritional status, and athlete body fat content. Although sex hormone receptors are found on ACL tissue, currently no direct molecular mechanisms of rupture have been identified.

Rupture incidence during the ovulatory cycle is greatest during the preovulatory phase[11] at 9 to 14 days[1] and declines as the menstrual cycle progresses.[26,27] Our current understanding of the effect of cycle-dependent changes in ligament mechanical characteristics is not clear. Although during the midpoint of the menstrual cycle the ACL does seem to have 0.5 mm more laxity, this is just the opposite of most data citing increased tear rates during the preovulatory phase.[28,29] The significance of this relationship is not well understood. It is possible that decreased ligament compliance in the preovulatory phase could contribute to the higher tear rate. However, it is possible that the increased tear rates seen during the preovulatory phase are due to changes in neuromuscular control and muscle contractility and not due to changes in the mechanical properties of the ACL.

In fact, the greatest effect of hormone influence on ACL rupture is most likely due to differences in neuromuscular growth and maturation during puberty rather than through direct effects on the ligament. Despite large increases in female height and weight during puberty, relatively low surges in testosterone in girls result in less strength gain relative to boys. This lower strength gain may be the cause of the neuro-muscular deficits and imbalances witnessed in ACL–at-risk athletes, with girls using ligaments and bone structure to modulate joint motion instead of muscle strength during activity.

Finally, external factors, such as footwear, playing surface, and type of competition, may contribute to sex nonparity in ACL rupture. Higher cleat number and artificial turf pitches increase the coefficient of friction and rate of ACL injury.[30,31]

PREVENTION OF ANTERIOR CRUCIATE LIGAMENT TEAR

Given the mounting evidence that ACL rupture results from repetitive biomechanical stresses across the ACL due to deficits in the neuromuscular coordination of muscle and knee joint, there is a great interest in preventing ACL rupture by training young ath-letes. The goal is to improve muscle firing patterns and to enhance unconscious motor responses in the central nervous system to produce a state of muscle readiness, increase motor control, and dynamic stability.

No universal program currently exists; however, all programs should include hip and hamstring training, core stability, balance, agility, and verbal feedback on landing techniques.[32] Sugimoto preformed a meta-analysis of 14 neuromuscular training (NMT) studies including more than 23,000 athletes. The meta-analysis reviewed 7 level 1 trials looking at study design, sports, age, dosage, exercise, and verbal feedback. They found a significant reduction of ACL tears by 17.2% to 17.7%. Furthermore, they identified the critical components as younger age, NMT dosage greater than 20 minutes twice a week, greater exercise variation, and verbal cueing. Multiple studies found athletes participating in 6 weeks of preseason training focusing on plyo-metrics, weight training, and flexibility were 3.6 times less likely to sustain knee injury.[10,33–35]

These programs focus on the gluteal muscles as key protectors against knee valgus, with the gluteus medius keeping the hip in abduction in landing, cutting, and direction change. Gluteus maximus was also a key predictor of lower extremity injury.[36] The programs should include progressive core stability, hip and hamstring strength, functional exercises (for establishing neuromuscular control), calf training (to ensure critical ankle stability and postural control to stabilize the knee during decel-eration), learning how to absorb landing force/preventing knee buckling, as well as feedback-driven plyometric technique modification.[36–40]

Johnson and colleagues[41] found that training outcomes for youth athletes are related to their psychological resilience. This resilience can be modulated by constructive communication, rich interaction with significant family members, a strong belief in the importance and efficacy of their own actions, and learning to set reasonable goals.

Ideally, ACL prevention programs should consist of 15 to 18 target training sessions over 6 to 8 weeks at a frequency of 2 times per week both before season and in-season. These sessions should begin in the prepubertal period and be designed in an age and maturation-specific manner with a focus on NMT with fatigue resistance.[15]

Interestingly, ACL prevention programs have not been found to increase on-field speed and agility performance, thus, making adherence by coaches and athletes diffi-cult as there is not a dual benefit.[42] Hagglund and colleagues[43] found that coach-led training is most effective because of high compliance and resulted in fewer injuries in soccer.

CLINICAL MANAGEMENT

Most ACL injuries require surgical management in the form of ACL reconstruction, particularly in young, high-demand athletes. The key to achieving optimal outcomes is to approach ACL rupture management in a structured, evidence-based, yet individualized approach.[44,45] A thorough history and physical examination is paramount, and secondary stabilizers (such as menisci and collaterals) should be assessed for injury.

Once the decision is made to reconstruct the torn ACL, it is crucial to restore the patients' individual anatomy. This restoration includes matching the native femoral and tibial insertion sites, appropriate placement of bony tunnels, choosing the proper graft, and choosing the correct graft size. Although data have shown that grafts less than 8 mm in diameter are more likely to fail,[8,46,47] it is also possible to cause premature failure by using too large of a graft relative to femoral notch size. This large graft would cause impingement and, ultimately, rupture.[48] A substantial body of evidence has demonstrated that autograft is more reliable in young patients,[49,50] although the ideal autograft harvest site remains controversial.[51–55]

The bone-patellar tendon-bone graft has long been considered the gold standard. The benefit of its bone-to-bone healing is widely considered to result in faster graft incorporation and lower rerupture rates.[51] However, it usually requires a larger incision and is associated with an increased incidence of anterior knee pain. The hamstring tendon is one of the most popular options, requires only a small incision for harvest, and can readily be augmented with allograft to obtain a larger graft diameter,[56] if necessary. However, it takes longer to incorporate than grafts with a bone block[57]; some studies suggest a higher rerupture rate compared with bone-patellar tendon bone,[53] though most evidence shows no difference in outcomes between the two grafts. Some investigators have expressed concern about increased dynamic knee valgus instability after hamstring harvest, but clinical outcomes have not shown a difference. A third, though less used option, is the quad tendon. It is not associated with anterior knee pain,[54] has higher collagen density and surface area than bone-patellar tendon-bone, and has been associated with low failure rates.[58] The downsides to this approach include a less cosmetically pleasing scar from the harvest incision and there is often some degree of quad weakness in the initial postoperative phase.

High-grade rotatory instability requires additional consideration of abnormal bony morphology, meniscal injury, posterior menisco-capsular injury, anterolateral complex injury, generalized joint laxity, and other potential contributors to this instability.[59–65] In some cases, extra-articular reconstruction procedures may be needed, although the proper indications and long-term effects of these procedures are poorly understood.[66–71] Tibial-slope altering osteotomies may be indicated in patients with extremely high tibial slopes, although this procedure is usually reserved for revision cases.[72]

Although many surgical variations, graft choices, and technique differences in ACL reconstruction exist, restoration of the native ACL anatomy, utilization of autograft in young and active patients, identification of concomitant injuries, and individualization of the surgery according to specific patients' anatomy and functional demands will help maximize the chances of success.

RETURN TO SPORT

Optimal return-to-sport (RTS) guidelines after ACL reconstruction are well studied, yet poorly understood. Several components must be considered, including chronologic time from surgery; neuromuscular performance, including quad, hamstring, hip, and trunk strength; as well as psychological factors, including kinesophobia and patient hardiness.[4,39,73–77] Unfortunately, no single test can assess RTS readiness, and no single battery of tests is agreed on.

Time is an important consideration in RTS assessment. ACL reconstruction grafts undergo ligamentization, whereby they are incorporated into the native ACL site and undergo changes that result in a more similar histologic and structural appearance to the native ACL. However, reconstructed grafts never achieve the same strength, vascularity, or innervation as the native ACL. Furthermore, rehabilitation protocols were initially developed based on animal studies of ACL graft ligamentization. Human studies have demonstrated that, although the ligamentization process is similar to animals, it likely takes much longer in humans and the graft may not achieve optimal structural characteristics for more than 1 year after surgery.[57,78,79]

Neuromuscular control and muscular strength are key factors in RTS. Although the importance of quad and hamstring strength to ACL rehabilitation are well known, hip and core strength have recently been shown to predict noncontact ACL injury.[80,81] The impact of hip, core, and trunk strength on ACL injury risk is even more robust in female athletes, as studies have shown more risky landing and cutting mechanics in females.[1,82] As the influence of the hip and trunk in the ACL injury mechanism is better understood, it is important to target rehabilitation efforts to treat these deficits and to use screening tests that can accurately gauge hip, core, and trunk function. Although many functional tests have been proposed, the single-leg hop tests, the single-leg step-down test (**Fig. 1**), and the Y-balance test (**Fig. 2**) have shown particular utility

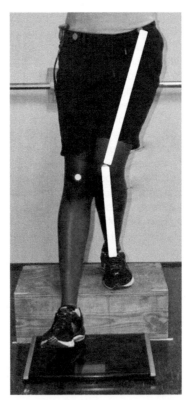

Fig. 1. Single-leg step-down test. Note the dynamic knee valgus of the stance leg, indicating weak hip musculature, suggestive of increased ACL injury risk.

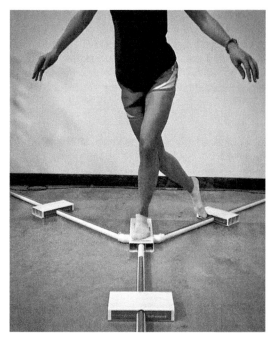

Fig. 2. Y-balance test. The subject's maximum reach distance in the anterior, posteromedial, and posterolateral directions is recorded; comparison of these values with the contralateral limb can predict lower extremity injury risk.

in the setting of ACL RTS testing.[37,78,83–85] Although the limb symmetry index (LSI) has been traditionally used to judge RTS readiness (85%–90% functional test performance compared with the uninjured limb), recent data have suggested that the uninjured extremity may exhibit postsurgical deficits; thus, the LSI must be interpreted with caution.

Even on completion of functional rehabilitation programs, motor deficits may persist, plaguing athletes with the same motor patterns that predisposed them to injury in the first place. Neuromuscular deficits may persist even 12 months after an ACL reconstruction; however, these deficits can be modulated by 6 weeks of kettle bell training for hamstring activation[86] and trunk control.[87] Hewett and colleagues[82] summarized the data on neuromuscular training programs and suggested that NMT programs most effectively decrease ACL injuries if they (1) include "plyometrics, balance, and strengthening exercises," (2) are performed more than once per week, and (3) are performed for a minimum of 6 weeks.

Another important but often overlooked component of RTS readiness is patients' psychological health. Several studies have demonstrated the importance of mental health on outcomes after musculoskeletal injury.[88–92] Furthermore, psychological traits, such as pain catastrophizing,[92] hardiness,[89] and kinesophobia,[90] have been linked to outcomes after ACL reconstruction, especially in younger patients. Therefore, it is important to consider the psychological state of ACL reconstruction patients and provide appropriate intervention when necessary.[41]

SUMMARY

The incidence of ACL rupture in female athletes is steadily increasing. As females continue to become more engaged in high-level and competitive sports, this trend is unlikely to change. Therapists, athletic trainers, coaches, and physicians must remain vigilant in implementing preventative NMT programs, effective screening tests, and appropriate treatment and rehabilitation when ACL rupture does occur. Although current knowledge and techniques have advanced significantly over the last decade, there remains ample opportunity to improve the outcomes of female athletes relative to ACL injury risk and rehabilitation.

REFERENCES

1. Arendt EA. Musculoskeletal injuries of the knee: are females at greater risk? Minn Med 2007;90(6):38–40.
2. Renstrom P, Ljungqvist A, Arendt E, et al. Non-contact ACL injuries in female athletes: an International Olympic Committee current concepts statement. Br J Sports Med 2008;42(6):394–412.
3. Snaebjornsson T, Hamrin Senorski E, Sundemo D, et al. Adolescents and female patients are at increased risk for contralateral anterior cruciate ligament reconstruction: a cohort study from the Swedish National Knee Ligament Register based on 17,682 patients. Knee Surg Sports Traumatol Arthrosc 2017. [Epub ahead of print].
4. Paterno MV, Rauh MJ, Schmitt LC, et al. Incidence of second ACL injuries 2 years after primary ACL reconstruction and return to sport. Am J Sports Med 2014; 42(7):1567–73.
5. Brophy R, Silvers HJ, Gonzales T, et al. Gender influences: the role of leg dominance in ACL injury among soccer players. Br J Sports Med 2010;44(10):694–7.
6. Brophy RH, Schmitz L, Wright RW, et al. Return to play and future ACL injury risk after ACL reconstruction in soccer athletes from the Multicenter Orthopaedic Outcomes Network (MOON) group. Am J Sports Med 2012;40(11):2517–22.
7. Soderman K, Pietila T, Alfredson H, et al. Anterior cruciate ligament injuries in young females playing soccer at senior levels. Scand J Med Sci Sports 2002; 12(2):65–8.
8. Nguyen D. Sex, age, and graft size as predictors of ACL re-tear: a multivariate logistic regression of a cohort of 503 athletes. Orthop J Sports Med 2016; 4(7 Suppl):2325967116S00164.
9. Allen MM, Pareek A, Krych AJ, et al. Are female soccer players at an increased risk of second anterior cruciate ligament injury compared with their athletic peers? Am J Sports Med 2016;44(10):2492–8.
10. Bukoskey TP, Graves M, Humphreys R. Relationship between prophylactic management of predisposing risk factors and noncontact ACL injuries with female athletes: analysis of the evidence-based literature. J Natl Soc Allied Health 2010;7(8):17–25.
11. Wojtys EM. The ACL dilemma. Sports Health 2012;4(1):12–3.
12. Trentacosta NE, Vitale MA, Ahmad CS. The effects of timing of pediatric knee ligament surgery on short-term academic performance in school-aged athletes. Am J Sports Med 2009;37(9):1684–91.
13. Swenson DM, Collins CL, Best TM, et al. Epidemiology of knee injuries among U.S. high school athletes, 2005/2006-2010/2011. Med Sci Sports Exerc 2013; 45(3):462–9.
14. Hagglund M, Walden M. Risk factors for acute knee injury in female youth football. Knee Surg Sports Traumatol Arthrosc 2016;24(3):737–46.

15. De Ste Croix MB, Priestley AM, Lloyd RS, et al. ACL injury risk in elite female youth soccer: changes in neuromuscular control of the knee following soccer-specific fatigue. (1600-0838 (Electronic)). Scand J Med Sci Sports 2015;25(5):e531–8.

16. Myer GD, Brent JL, Ford KR, et al. Real-time assessment and neuromuscular training feedback techniques to prevent ACL injury in female athletes. Strength Cond J 2011;33(3):21–35.

17. Pfeiffer RP, Shea KG, Roberts D, et al. Lack of effect of a knee ligament injury prevention program on the incidence of noncontact anterior cruciate ligament injury. J Bone Joint Surg Am 2006;88(8):1769–74.

18. Leppanen M, Pasanen K, Kulmala JP, et al. Knee control and jump-landing technique in young basketball and floorball players. Int J Sports Med 2016;37(4): 334–8.

19. Chappell JD, Yu B, Kirkendall DT, et al. A comparison of knee kinetics between male and female recreational athletes in stop-jump tasks. Am J Sports Med 2002;30(2):261–7.

20. Loudon JK, Jenkins W, Loudon KL. The relationship between static posture and ACL injury in female athletes. J Orthop Sports Phys Ther 1996;24(2):91–7.

21. Pappas E, Shiyko MP, Ford KR, et al. Biomechanical deficit profiles associated with ACL injury risk in female athletes. Med Sci Sports Exerc 2016;48(1):107–13.

22. Chandrashekar N, Mansouri H, Slauterbeck J, et al. Sex-based differences in the tensile properties of the human anterior cruciate ligament. J Biomech 2006; 39(16):2943–50.

23. Stijak L, Blagojevic Z, Santrac-Stijak G, et al. Predicting ACL rupture in the population actively engaged in sports activities based on anatomical risk factors. Orthopedics 2011;34(6):431.

24. Sturnick DR, Van Gorder R, Vacek PM, et al. Tibial articular cartilage and meniscus geometries combine to influence female risk of anterior cruciate ligament injury. J Orthop Res 2014;32(11):1487–94.

25. Beynnon BD, Hall JS, Sturnick DR, et al. Increased slope of the lateral tibial plateau subchondral bone is associated with greater risk of noncontact ACL injury in females but not in males: a prospective cohort study with a nested, matched case-control analysis. Am J Sports Med 2014;42(5):1039–48.

26. Ruedl G, Ploner P, Linortner I, et al. Are oral contraceptive use and menstrual cycle phase related to anterior cruciate ligament injury risk in female recreational skiers? Knee Surg Sports Traumatol Arthrosc 2009;17(9):1065–9.

27. Slauterbeck JR, Fuzie SF, Smith MP, et al. The menstrual cycle, sex hormones, and anterior cruciate ligament injury. J Athl Train 2002;37(3):275–8.

28. Hewett TE, Zazulak BT, Myer GD. Effects of the menstrual cycle on anterior cruciate ligament injury risk: a systematic review. Am J Sports Med 2007;35(4): 659–68.

29. Wojtys EM, Huston LJ, Lindenfeld TN, et al. Association between the menstrual cycle and anterior cruciate ligament injuries in female athletes. Am J Sports Med 1998;26(5):614–9.

30. Lambson RB, Barnhill BS, Higgins RW. Football cleat design and its effect on anterior cruciate ligament injuries. A three-year prospective study. Am J Sports Med 1996;24(2):155–9.

31. Olsen OE, Myklebust G, Engebretsen L, et al. Relationship between floor type and risk of ACL injury in team handball. Scand J Med Sci Sports 2003;13(5): 299–304.

32. Bien DP. Rationale and implementation of anterior cruciate ligament injury prevention warm-up programs in female athletes. J Strength Cond Res 2011;25(1): 271–85.

33. Myer GD, Ford KR, Palumbo JP, et al. Neuromuscular training improves performance and lower-extremity biomechanics in female athletes. J Strength Cond Res 2005;19(1):51–60.

34. Taylor JB, Waxman JP, Richter SJ, et al. Evaluation of the effectiveness of anterior cruciate ligament injury prevention programme training components: a systematic review and meta-analysis. Br J Sports Med 2015;49(2):79–87.

35. Grimm NL, Jacobs JC Jr, Kim J, et al. Anterior cruciate ligament and knee injury prevention programs for soccer players: a systematic review and meta-analysis. Am J Sports Med 2015;43(8):2049–56.

36. Leetun DT, Ireland ML, Willson JD, et al. Core stability measures as risk factors for lower extremity injury in athletes. Med Sci Sports Exerc 2004;36(6):926–34.

37. Burnham JM, Yonz MC, Robertson KE, et al. Relationship of hip and trunk muscle function with single leg step-down performance: implications for return to play screening and rehabilitation. Phys Ther Sport 2016;22:66–73.

38. Griffin LY, Agel J, Albohm MJ, et al. Noncontact anterior cruciate ligament injuries: risk factors and prevention strategies. J Am Acad Orthop Surg 2000;8(3):141–50.

39. Kline PW, Johnson DL, Ireland ML, et al. Clinical predictors of knee mechanics at return to sport after ACL reconstruction. Med Sci Sports Exerc 2016;48(5):790–5.

40. Willson JD, Dougherty CP, Ireland ML, et al. Core stability and its relationship to lower extremity function and injury. J Am Acad Orthop Surg 2005;13(5):316–25.

41. Johnson U, Ivarsson A, Karlsson J, et al. Rehabilitation after first-time anterior cruciate ligament injury and reconstruction in female football players: a study of resilience factors. BMC Sports Sci Med Rehabil 2016;8:20.

42. Vescovi JD, VanHeest JL. Effects of an anterior cruciate ligament injury prevention program on performance in adolescent female soccer players. Scand J Med Sci Sports 2010;20(3):394–402.

43. Hagglund M, Atroshi I, Wagner P, et al. Superior compliance with a neuromuscular training programme is associated with fewer ACL injuries and fewer acute knee injuries in female adolescent football players: secondary analysis of an RCT. Br J Sports Med 2013;47(15):974–9.

44. Araujo PH, Kfuri Junior M, Ohashi B, et al. Individualized ACL reconstruction. Knee Surg Sports Traumatol Arthrosc 2014;22(9):1966–75.

45. Rabuck SJ, Middleton KK, Maeda S, et al. Individualized anatomic anterior cruciate ligament reconstruction. Arthrosc Tech 2012;1(1):e23–9.

46. Mariscalco MW, Flanigan DC, Mitchell J, et al. The influence of hamstring autograft size on patient-reported outcomes and risk of revision after anterior cruciate ligament reconstruction: a Multicenter Orthopaedic Outcomes Network (MOON) cohort study. Arthroscopy 2013;29(12):1948–53.

47. Magnussen RA, Lawrence JT, West RL, et al. Graft size and patient age are predictors of early revision after anterior cruciate ligament reconstruction with hamstring autograft. Arthroscopy 2012;28(4):526–31.

48. Gormeli CA, Gormeli G, Ozturk BY, et al. The effect of the intercondylar notch width index on anterior cruciate ligament injuries: a study on groups with unilateral and bilateral ACL injury. Acta Orthop Belg 2015;81(2):240–4.

49. Engelman GH, Carry PM, Hitt KG, et al. Comparison of allograft versus autograft anterior cruciate ligament reconstruction graft survival in an active adolescent cohort. Am J Sports Med 2014;42(10):2311–8.

50. Rice RS, Waterman BR, Lubowitz JH. Allograft versus autograft decision for anterior cruciate ligament reconstruction: an expected-value decision analysis evaluating hypothetical patients. Arthroscopy 2012;28(4):539–47.

51. Gabler CM, Jacobs CA, Howard JS, et al. Comparison of graft failure rate between autografts placed via an anatomic anterior cruciate ligament reconstruction technique: a systematic review, meta-analysis, and meta-regression. Am J Sports Med 2016;44(4):1069–79.

52. Rahr-Wagner L, Thillemann TM, Pedersen AB, et al. Comparison of hamstring tendon and patellar tendon grafts in anterior cruciate ligament reconstruction in a nationwide population-based cohort study: results from the Danish registry of knee ligament reconstruction. Am J Sports Med 2014;42(2):278–84.

53. Persson A, Fjeldsgaard K, Gjertsen JE, et al. Increased risk of revision with hamstring tendon grafts compared with patellar tendon grafts after anterior cruciate ligament reconstruction: a study of 12,643 patients from the Norwegian Cruciate Ligament Registry, 2004-2012. Am J Sports Med 2014;42(2):285–91.

54. Buescu CT, Onutu AH, Lucaciu DO, et al. Pain level after ACL reconstruction: a comparative study between free quadriceps tendon and hamstring tendons autografts. Acta Orthop Traumatol Turc 2017;51(2):100–3.

55. Mohtadi N, Chan D, Barber R, et al. A randomized clinical trial comparing patellar tendon, hamstring tendon, and double-bundle ACL reconstructions: patient-reported and clinical outcomes at a minimal 2-year follow-up. Clin J Sport Med 2015;25(4):321–31.

56. Jacobs CA, Burnham JM, Makhni E, et al. Allograft augmentation of hamstring autograft for younger patients undergoing anterior cruciate ligament reconstruction. Am J Sports Med 2017;45(4):892–9.

57. Ma Y, Murawski CD, Rahnemai-Azar AA, et al. Graft maturity of the reconstructed anterior cruciate ligament 6 months postoperatively: a magnetic resonance imaging evaluation of quadriceps tendon with bone block and hamstring tendon autografts. Knee Surg Sports Traumatol Arthrosc 2015;23(3):661–8.

58. Cavaignac E, Coulin B, Tscholl P, et al. Is quadriceps tendon autograft a better choice than hamstring autograft for anterior cruciate ligament reconstruction? A comparative study with a mean follow-up of 3.6 years. Am J Sports Med 2017; 45(6):1326–32.

59. Rahnemai-Azar AA, Zlotnicki J, Burnham JM, et al. Secondary stabilizers of the anterior cruciate ligament—deficient knee. Oper Tech Orthop 2017;27(2):107–12.

60. Herbst E, Albers M, Burnham JM, et al. The anterolateral complex of the knee: a pictorial essay. Knee Surg Sports Traumatol Arthrosc 2017;25(4):1009–14.

61. Burnham JM, Herbst E, Pauyo T, et al. Technical considerations in revision anterior cruciate ligament reconstruction for operative techniques in orthopaedics. Oper Tech Orthop 2017;27(1):63–9.

62. Rahnemai-Azar AA, Yaseen Z, van Eck CF, et al. Increased lateral tibial plateau slope predisposes male college football players to anterior cruciate ligament injury. J Bone Joint Surg Am 2016;98(12):1001–6.

63. Rahnemai-Azar AA, Abebe ES, Johnson P, et al. Increased lateral tibial slope predicts high-grade rotatory knee laxity pre-operatively in ACL reconstruction. Knee Surg Sports Traumatol Arthrosc 2017;25(4):1170–6.

64. Musahl V, Rahnemai-Azar AA, Costello J, et al. The influence of meniscal and anterolateral capsular injury on knee laxity in patients with anterior cruciate ligament injuries. Am J Sports Med 2016;44(12):3126–31.

65. Arner J, Herbst E, Burnham JM, et al. MRI can accurately detect meniscal ramp lesions of the knee. Knee Surg Sports Traumatol Arthrosc 2017. [Epub ahead of print].

66. Noyes FR, Huser LE, Levy MS. Rotational knee instability in ACL-deficient knees: role of the anterolateral ligament and iliotibial band as defined by tibiofemoral compartment translations and rotations. J Bone Joint Surg Am 2017;99(4): 305–14.

67. Sonnery-Cottet B, Lutz C, Daggett M, et al. The involvement of the anterolateral ligament in rotational control of the knee. Am J Sports Med 2016;44(5):1209–14.

68. Sonnery-Cottet B, Daggett M, Helito CP, et al. Combined anterior cruciate ligament and anterolateral ligament reconstruction. Arthrosc Tech 2016;5(6): e1253–9.

69. Shea KG, Polousky JD, Jacobs JC Jr, et al. The anterolateral ligament of the knee: an inconsistent finding in pediatric cadaveric specimens. J Pediatr Orthop 2016; 36(5):e51–4.

70. Schon JM, Moatshe G, Brady AW, et al. Anatomic anterolateral ligament reconstruction of the knee leads to overconstraint at any fixation angle. Am J Sports Med 2016;44(10):2546–56.

71. Musahl V, Getgood A, Neyret P, et al. Contributions of the anterolateral complex and the anterolateral ligament to rotatory knee stability in the setting of ACL injury: a roundtable discussion. Knee Surg Sports Traumatol Arthrosc 2017;25(4): 997–1008.

72. Won HH, Chang CB, Je MS, et al. Coronal limb alignment and indications for high tibial osteotomy in patients undergoing revision ACL reconstruction. Clin Orthop Relat Res 2013;471(11):3504–11.

73. Sonesson S, Kvist J, Ardern C, et al. Psychological factors are important to return to pre-injury sport activity after anterior cruciate ligament reconstruction: expect and motivate to satisfy. Knee Surg Sports Traumatol Arthrosc 2017;25(5): 1375–84.

74. Howard JS, Lembach ML, Metzler AV, et al. Rates and determinants of return to play after anterior cruciate ligament reconstruction in National Collegiate Athletic Association Division I soccer athletes: a study of the Southeastern Conference. Am J Sports Med 2016;44(2):433–9.

75. Mayer SW, Queen RM, Taylor D, et al. Functional testing differences in anterior cruciate ligament reconstruction patients released versus not released to return to sport. Am J Sports Med 2015;43(7):1648–55.

76. Herbst E, Hoser C, Hildebrandt C, et al. Functional assessments for decision-making regarding return to sports following ACL reconstruction. Part II: clinical application of a new test battery. Knee Surg Sports Traumatol Arthrosc 2015; 23(5):1283–91.

77. Shelbourne KD, Benner RW, Gray T. Return to sports and subsequent injury rates after revision anterior cruciate ligament reconstruction with patellar tendon autograft. Am J Sports Med 2014;42(6):1395–400.

78. Joreitz R, Lynch A, Rabuck S, et al. Patient-specific and surgery-specific factors that affect return to sport after ACL reconstruction. Int J Sports Phys Ther 2016; 11(2):264–78.

79. Janssen RP, Scheffler SU. Intra-articular remodelling of hamstring tendon grafts after anterior cruciate ligament reconstruction. Knee Surg Sports Traumatol Arthrosc 2014;22(9):2102–8.

80. Khayambashi K, Ghoddosi N, Straub RK, et al. Hip muscle strength predicts noncontact anterior cruciate ligament injury in male and female athletes: a prospective study. Am J Sports Med 2016;44(2):355–61.
81. Brumitt J, Heiderscheit BC, Manske RC, et al. Lower extremity functional tests and risk of injury in division iii collegiate athletes. Int J Sports Phys Ther 2013; 8(3):216–27.
82. Hewett TE, Ford KR, Myer GD. Anterior cruciate ligament injuries in female athletes: part 2, a meta-analysis of neuromuscular interventions aimed at injury prevention. Am J Sports Med 2006;34(3):490–8.
83. Lee DK, Kim GM, Ha SM, et al. Correlation of the Y-balance test with lower-limb strength of adult women. J Phys Ther Sci 2014;26(5):641–3.
84. Shirey M, Hurlbutt M, Johansen N, et al. The influence of core musculature engagement on hip and knee kinematics in women during a single leg squat. Int J Sports Phys Ther 2012;7(1):1–12.
85. Xergia SA, Pappas E, Zampeli F, et al. Asymmetries in functional hop tests, lower extremity kinematics, and isokinetic strength persist 6 to 9 months following anterior cruciate ligament reconstruction. J Orthop Sports Phys Ther 2013;43(3): 154–62.
86. Zebis MK, Andersen CH, Bencke J, et al. Neuromuscular coordination deficit persists 12 months after ACL reconstruction but can be modulated by 6 weeks of kettlebell training: a case study in women's elite soccer. Case Rep Orthop 2017;2017:4269575.
87. Noehren B, Abraham A, Curry M, et al. Evaluation of proximal joint kinematics and muscle strength following ACL reconstruction surgery in female athletes. J Orthop Res 2014;32(10):1305–10.
88. Wylie JD, Suter T, Potter MQ, et al. Mental health has a stronger association with patient-reported shoulder pain and function than tear size in patients with full-thickness rotator cuff tears. J Bone Joint Surg Am 2016;98(4):251–6.
89. Salim J, Wadey R, Diss C. Examining hardiness coping and stress related growth following sport injury. J Appl Sport Psychol 2015;28(2):154–69.
90. Hartigan EH, Lynch AD, Logerstedt DS, et al. Kinesiophobia after anterior cruciate ligament rupture and reconstruction: noncopers versus potential copers. J Orthop Sports Phys Ther 2013;43(11):821–32.
91. Hamdan TA. Psychiatric aspects of orthopaedics. J Am Acad Orthop Surg 2008; 16(1):41–6.
92. Tripp DA, Stanish WD, Reardon G, et al. Comparing postoperative pain experiences of the adolescent and adult athlete after anterior cruciate ligament surgery. J Athl Train 2003;38(2):154–7.

Sport Concussion and the Female Athlete

Jacob E. Resch, PhD[a],*, Amanda Rach, PhD[b], Samuel Walton, MEd[a],
Donna K. Broshek, PhD[b]

KEYWORDS

• Neurocognitive • Hormone • Concussion • Sex differences

KEY POINTS

• Current evidence is mixed regarding sex differences in cognitive performance after a sport concussion (SC).

• Female athletes have a higher symptom burden before and after injury, which should be accounted for when making evidence-based decisions regarding SC.

• Female athletes have been routinely observed to have increased risk for SC, which may be partially explained by physical and physiologic differences.

• In terms of protracted recovery after an SC, the data remain equivocal; regardless of biological sex, athletes diagnosed with an SC should be managed based on clinical presentation.

INTRODUCTION

In 2016, a survey-based study asked the question, "Would you let your child play football?"[1] Given the popularity of American football and that it is primarily a male sport, the title of this study emphasized the incidence and cumulative effects of sport concussion (SC) in male athletes. Since 1999,[2] an increasing body of literature has reported that female athletes who participate in sports with a male counterpart (eg, softball vs baseball) have an equal if not increased risk of SC. Despite awareness of female athletes' increased susceptibility to injury[3] and postconcussion symptom reporting,[4] as well as decreased neurocognitive[5] and balance performance,[4] SC-related research attention is primarily focused on male athletes. Our current knowledge of specific risk factors and outcomes related to SC and the female athlete compels additional questions about the risk(s) associated with female participation in contact and noncontact sports.

[a] Department of Kinesiology, University of Virginia, 210 Emmet Street South, Charlottesville, VA 22904, USA; [b] Department of Psychiatry and Neurobehavioral Sciences, University of Virginia School of Medicine, 1300 Jefferson Park Avenue, Charlottesville, VA 22908, USA
* Corresponding author.
E-mail address: jer6x@virginia.edu

Clin Sports Med 36 (2017) 717–739
http://dx.doi.org/10.1016/j.csm.2017.05.002
0278-5919/17/© 2017 Elsevier Inc. All rights reserved.

sportsmed.theclinics.com

EPIDEMIOLOGY

When all sports are considered, epidemiologic studies of SC within the last 2 decades have demonstrated that male athletes sustain more concussions than female athletes.[2,3,6–23] However, when considering female sports with a male equivalent (eg, basketball and soccer), female athletes sustain more SCs compared with male athletes. **Fig. 1** summarizes published SC injury rates (IR) between male and female sports.[3,6,8,10]

Overall, male high school and collegiate athletes have been found to have a higher SC rate than female athletes.[6,7,9] However, when considering male sports with an equivalent female counterpart, high school and collegiate females have an equal or higher rate of SC compared with males.[3,6,8,10] Based on data collected by the National Collegiate Athletic Association Surveillance System between the 1988 and 1989 sports seasons, only 1 study indicated a higher SC rate for males (IR = 45 per 100,000 athletic exposures [AEs]) compared with females (IR = 38 per 100,000 AEs) for all sports.[9] The discrepancy between this study compared with the majority of investigations was due to the inclusion of football and wrestling in addition to other male sports. In contrast, when all secondary school and collegiate female sports were considered, SC rates ranged between 13 and 38[6,7,9] per 100,000 AEs. For high school and collegiate male sports, reported IR have ranged between 25 and 45 per 100,000 AEs.[6,7,9] In summary, the epidemiologic evidence suggests that female athletes who participate in a sport with a male counterpart have an equal if not increased risk of sustaining an SC.

PHYSICAL AND PHYSIOLOGIC ASPECTS OF THE FEMALE ATHLETE AND CONCUSSION
Neck Strength

One plausible reason for the previously discussed increased incidence of SC in female sports is neck strength. Early studies that examined sex differences in terms of neck

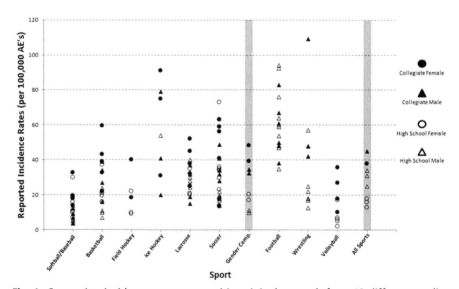

Fig. 1. Concussion incidence rates reported in original research from 19 different studies; athletic years 1997 to 2015 in collegiate athletes (11 studies) and 1995 to 2014 in high school athletes (15 studies). AE, athlete exposure, defined as one athlete participating in a single game or practice; All Sports, all sports for each sex as reported by each study that calculated this as a separate comparison; Gender Comp., gender comparable sports as reported by each study that calculated this as a separate comparison. (*Data from* Refs.[2,7–9,11–25])

strength focused on head–neck segment mass and dynamic stabilization, which is defined as the ability of a myotendon unit to absorb external loads and minimize excessive joint movement.[24] Tierney and colleagues[24] compared 20 collegiate males with 20 collegiate females in terms of head–neck segment anthropometrics, kinematics, and neuromuscular control via electromyography. Participants were equipped with head gear connected to a pulley system, which allowed for a 1-kg mass to be dropped 15 cm. Female participants had up to 43% less head–neck segment mass and exhibited 25% more angular acceleration compared with male subjects. This finding is similar to related studies that reported female athlete neck strength was negatively correlated ($r = -0.50$ to -0.76) with linear acceleration, whereas heading soccer balls propelled at speeds up to 40 miles per hour.[25,26] Additionally, Tierney and colleagues reported female participants exhibited 50% less isometric strength and up to 117% more muscle activity as recorded via electromyography compared with male subjects. The authors concluded female athletes may be predisposed to SC resulting from a decreased head–neck segment mass, leading to an increased angular velocity after potential concussive impact.[27]

In a separate study, Tierney and colleagues[27] examined sex differences in terms of the same variables with the addition of linear acceleration while heading a soccer ball with and without head gear. Similar to their previous study, female subjects were observed to have significantly less head–neck segment mass and isometric neck strength and a significantly greater amount of muscle activity compared with male participants. In terms of linear acceleration, females were observed to have up to a 32% (~ 5 g) increase in linear acceleration when wearing headgear and a 10% increase (~ 2 g) without. In addition to the anthropometric and kinematic sex differences, a unique finding of this study was that female participants donning protective head gear sustained greater linear acceleration forces compared with males with and without headgear.[27] Collins and colleagues[28] identified overall mean neck strength as a predictor of SCs in female athletes, which supports previous findings that decreased head–neck segment mass and isometric strength result in decreased head–neck stability and increased head–neck acceleration, predisposing female athletes to SC. Overall, these findings support the need for prospective research addressing the effects of neck-strengthening programs to reduce the likelihood of SC in female athletes.

Hormonal Considerations

Hormonal factors specific to female athletes have been demonstrated to be related to poor outcomes after SC. Alterations in pituitary function have been well-documented in both males and females who sustained a moderate or severe traumatic brain injury (TBI).[29–34] More specifically, TBI may result in a direct mechanical insult to the pituitary gland or an interruption of its blood supply via compression of the long and/or short hypophyseal portal veins.[29] Either disruption may result in deficiencies in one or more pituitary hormones including the gonadotrophins.[35] The gonadotrophins consist of luteinizing hormone and follicle-stimulating hormone, which are related directly to the production of progesterone and estrogen from cholesterol in the ovarian follicle and corpus luteum.[36] Progesterone and estrogen are suspected to have a neuroprotective effect for the prevention of mild TBI (mTBI)/SC.[37] Disruption of the hypothalamic–pituitary–gonadal axis as a result of the mechanical strain[38,39] and corresponding hemodynamic changes[40] after TBI may result in alterations in progesterone and estrogen synthesis and release, leading to poor outcomes after a concussion.

Female athletes have been reported to have increased symptom reporting,[4,37] time removed from normal activities (eg, work and sport), and greater cognitive deficits when compared with males, although the data for the latter finding are mixed.[3,37,41] Pertinent to SC is the timing of an injury in relation to a female's menstrual cycle because progesterone levels vary between luteal (high) and follicular phases (low). A preliminary study by Wunderle and colleagues[42] investigated the influence of menstrual cycle phase on 1-month quality of life and self-report symptom outcomes in female patients (16–60 years of age) who were diagnosed with concussion. Participants were grouped based on progesterone level, which was indicative of menstrual cycle phase (eg, luteal phase, follicular phase, and synthetic progesterone groups) at the time of admission to an emergency department. Their results supported a disruption in the hypothalamic–pituitary–gonadal axis as a result of concussion because females in the luteal phase (high levels of progesterone) experienced worse outcomes than participants in either the follicular phase (low levels of progesterone) or the synthetic progesterone (constant levels of progesterone) groups. The authors concluded that their data supported the "withdrawal hypothesis," in which females in the luteal phase at the time of their injury experienced a sudden decrease in progesterone, which was related to both result in lower quality of life ratings and higher symptom burden than females who already had a low or constant progesterone levels (ie, follicular and synthetic groups).[42] These data support previous studies that associated less precise measures of menstrual phase (premenstrual [luteal phase] vs menstrual period [follicular phase]) and use of contraceptives in terms of SC outcomes and risk.[43,44] The relation between mechanical strain and hemodynamic changes, as well as between hormones and timing of injury, as a possible explanation for female athletes' increased risk of an SC and potential poorer outcomes must be elucidated more fully before making evidence-based recommendations for clinical practice.

Neuroimaging

Studies using conventional neuroimaging (ie, computed tomography or MRI) generally concluded that SCs were not associated with structural brain changes and, as such, computed tomography or MRI scans are generally not recommended by SC management position papers as an aspect of diagnostic or management after an SC.[45–48] Concussions are conceptualized as a complex neurochemical cascade and increasingly sensitive imaging technologies (ie, diffusion-weighted MRI, magnetic resonance spectroscopy, and functional MRI) are better suited to examine the transient physiologic and chemical abnormalities that occur after a concussive injury.[49] Investigations using these techniques have found acute and persistent white matter changes after cumulative subconcussive injuries, as well as an SC.[50–52] Studies of female athletes with a history of SC compared with female athletes without a history of SCs have found microstructural alterations in the hippocampi, primary motor cortices of the frontal lobes, and corpus callosum, with these structural difference often found in females who had experienced multiple previous concussions, as opposed to only a single SC.[49,53] There is also emerging evidence that indicates that the physiologic cerebral changes are present on imaging even after the cognitive and physical symptoms have resolved, which may have significant implications for concussion management and return-to-play decisions in the future.

SPORT CONCUSSION MANAGEMENT
Baseline Assessment

The preinjury (baseline) assessment for SC has become a point of contention in the sports medicine community, regardless of athlete sex.[54–56] The baseline assessment typically consists of sideline and/or clinic-based measures of neurocognition, balance, and concussion-related symptomology and are acquired before the start of the academic/athletic year or an athlete's respective sport season. Data derived from the baseline assessment provide a means of comparison with data collected after an SC at variable time points (eg, within 24 hours of injury and/or upon an athlete reporting symptom free). These data are then used to complement the clinical examination and aid in clinical decision making. Additionally, the baseline assessment allows clinicians to account for premorbid variability such as the presence of attention deficit hyperactivity disorder, learning disorders,[57] psychiatric diagnoses,[58] and prior history of SC,[59–61] which have been demonstrated to influence neurocognitive, balance,[62,63] and symptom outcome scores.[64]

Individually administered, traditional paper-and-pencil neuropsychological tests have been found to be sensitive to the effects of an SC.[65,66] Each SC injury is unique and, thus, an assessment battery must measure the cognitive domains known to be affected by an SC injury while also accounting for the time-limited nature associated with athletics, which makes the traditional 4- to 6-hour comprehensive assessment impractical.[67] In general, an SC cognitive battery typically measures aspects of verbal and visual memory, processing speed, working memory, psychomotor speed, and executive functioning abilities.[67,68]

For example, one of the most well-known paper-and-pencil batteries is the Penn State test battery,[69] which includes the Hopkins Verbal Learning Test,[70] Symbol-Digit Modalities Test,[71] Trail Making Test,[72] Penn State Cancellation Test,[69] Controlled Oral Word Association,[73] Digit Span Test,[74] Stroop Color-Word Test,[75] and the Vigil Continuous Performance Test.[76]

The quality and value of data derived from the baseline assessment may be best determined by how it was obtained. Although best practices have not been well-established for clinical measures of balance or obtaining baseline symptoms, recommendations have been put forth in terms of the computerized neurocognitive test (CNT), which may translate to other clinical measures. Multiple factors can affect the integrity of CNT data, as well as the interpretation of the data, including technical hardware and software issues, data security, psychometric issues (reliability and validity), cultural or other individual athlete characteristics, and response validity.[77] Owing to increasing concerns about the misuse of baseline CNT, the American Academy of Clinical Neuropsychology and the National Academy of Neuropsychology issued a joint position paper in 2012 outlining position statements on the use of CNTs.[77] When conducting the baseline CNT, it has been suggested that no more than 10 athletes should be assessed at 1 time in a quiet environment to avoid potential distractions while completing the assessment.[78,79] Administering a CNT in a large group setting (>10 athletes) has been demonstrated to result in decreased neurocognitive performance and increased symptom reporting.[78,80] Clinicians must also be familiar with and/or trained to administer and interpret test findings. Covassin and colleagues[81] surveyed certified athletic trainers who used the Immediate Postconcussion Assessment and Cognitive Test (ImPACT) battery in their concussion management policy. Approximately 50% of certified athletic trainers reported not completing training specific to ImPACT and an equivalent number did not review individual baseline assessment results for validity.[81]

Another consideration of the baseline assessment is ensuring the equivalence of computer interface (ie, desktop computer) on which the CNT is administered across testing stations. Computer operating systems, software, web browser, type of mouse and keyboard, and computer type have been demonstrated to be a systematic source of error that may influence CNT performance.[82] Finally, clinicians must account for athlete effort while completing a preseason assessment. Purposeful underperformance or "sandbagging" on CNTs to return to play more quickly after an SC has arisen as a concern among the sports medicine community. Currently marketed CNTs have automated validity criteria that flag results suggestive of suboptimal effort or misunderstanding of test instructions. That said, it has been demonstrated that research participants who were instructed to intentionally sandbag still avoided being detected while providing a suboptimal effort.[83,84] To partially remedy this issue of suboptimal CNT performance, 1 or more clinicians are encouraged to proctor the completion of individual or group assessments and review each baseline assessment for inadequate effort.[79,82] A summary of these and other recommendations in terms of the completion of baseline CNT assessments may be found in **Table 1**.

The clinical usefulness of the baseline neurocognitive assessment has been brought into question. The financial and human resource implications have led to investigation of how premorbid assessment of neurocognitive function may or may not influence clinical decision making, patient outcomes and/or modify risk of SC.[55,56] Since 2000, large normative datasets have been established for CNTs. Some have recommended the use of these datasets in the absence of a baseline assessment to assist with clinical decision making after an SC.[55] Arnett and colleagues[85] presented a decision tree model with different rules for male and female athletes based on base rate data collected in their collegiate sport program over a 10-year period. In their model, they administer both CNTs and an abbreviated battery of paper-and-pencil tests. Analysis of preconcussion baseline data on 495 athletes revealed that fewer than 10% of male athletes had 5 or more borderline scores at baseline or 3 or more impaired scores, and fewer than 10% of female athletes had 3 or more borderline scores or 2 or more impaired scores. As a result, these authors suggest that in the

Table 1
Recommendations for concussion assessments

Administration[82]	Standardized techniques should be used to administer an assessment to minimize random and systematic error.
Environment[66–70]	When possible, dedicated devices and locations should be located in an environment with no or limited distractions.
Audio/visual settings[82]	For computerized testing: monitor brightness, contrast, resolution, position and displayed object size should be the same across testing stations. When applicable, headphones are preferred over speakers.
Group administration[80,81]	Groups consisting of <10 athletes are recommended to minimize distractions.
Proctoring[79–82]	Tests should be proctored by 1 or more trained clinicians. Proctors should control the external environment as well as monitor the behavior of the athlete, specifically regarding motivation and attention.
Quality control[79–81]	Neuropsychologists, clinicians and/or administrators should review all clinical measure outcomes scores to screen for suboptimal or invalid performance. Special considerations should be taken into account for modifying factors (such as attention deficit hyperactivity disorder or learning disability) to account for premorbid variability.
Repeatability[77,80,82]	Care should be taken to produce identical testing environments for all assessments to decrease extraneous sources of error on the assessment(s).

These recommendations were modified from computerized neurocognitive testing to be applicable to all concussion assessments.

absence of baseline data for comparison, 5 or more borderline scores in male athletes or 3 or more impaired scores after injury likely reflects the cognitive sequelae of concussion. Similarly, female athletes with 3 or more borderline scores or 2 or more impaired performances are likely demonstrating the cognitive effects of SC.

Because the evidence for use of normative data comparison is still in the formative phase of research, governing health care bodies including the National Athletic Trainers' Association advocate for the use of baseline neurocognitive assessment to assist in clinical decision making after an SC, especially to account for those with the aforementioned premorbid conditions, which may influence performance on neurocognitive measures.[45,48,54] For some athletes who are evaluated after SC, baseline cognitive data are not available for comparison. Further evidence is needed to elucidate the need for baseline assessments for the management of SC.

Sideline Measures of Sport Concussion

Since 1997, the sideline assessment of SC has advanced significantly with the introduction of standardized neurocognitive, balance and symptom measures. Upon a suspected on-the-field SC or more significant head and/or neck injury, an athletic trainer will perform a primary survey to rule out a more significant and potentially life-threatening injury (eg, cervical spine involvement, subdural or epidural bleeding), which requires emergent care and transport to a medical facility. After the completion of the primary survey, the athletic trainer will move the athlete to the sideline to complete the secondary survey and more thorough sideline evaluation. Before 1997, a variety of gross clinical measures of cognitive, balance, and symptoms were used to order to assess SC. In 1997, the Standardized Assessment of Concussion (SAC) was introduced as a brief and standardized neurocognitive assessment tool to evaluate SC.[86] The SAC contains sections that assess orientation, immediate memory, concentration, and delayed recall.[86] The SAC has been demonstrated to have weak to moderate test–retest reliability (intraclass correlation coefficient = 0.29–0.46) using varying test–retest intervals in young and collegiate athletes and high levels of sensitivity (95%) and specificity (76%) acutely after SC.[87–89]

Also during the late 1990s, an objective sideline measure of balance, the balance error scoring system (BESS), was introduced.[90] The BESS is a brief measure of postural stability for which athletes are asked to stand in a double leg, single leg, or tandem stance on both firm and foam surfaces.[90] Athletes are asked to remain in each stance with their hands on their iliac crests and their eyes closed for 20 seconds while an examiner counts the number of times the participant commits an error. BESS errors consist of opening of the eyes, moving 1 or both hands from the hips, stepping or stumbling, remaining out of a testing position for longer than 5 seconds, a participant moving their hip into more than 30° of flexion or abduction (single leg stance), and/or lifting the forefoot or heel. The BESS has been demonstrated to have moderate to strong intrarater (0.57–0.98), interrater (0.78–0.96), and test–retest (0.56–0.70) reliability with evidence of construct validity but limited evidence of sensitivity or specificity.[88–93]

In 2004, the SAC and BESS were combined with standardized clinical measures of symptomology, the Glasgow Coma Scale, and the Maddocks questions, and additional motor and neurocognitive tasks to form the standardized Sport Concussion Assessment Tool (SCAT).[94] In 2013, the third iteration of the SCAT was introduced along with the Child SCAT for the sideline evaluation of SC.[95] The clinical usefulness of various iterations of the SCAT has supported its use a sideline evaluation tool. Putukian and colleagues[89] demonstrated the SCAT 2 to have 96% sensitivity and 81% specificity when detecting the presence of an SC within 48 hours of injury. The authors also reported no premorbid or outcome differences between male and female athletes in terms of any outcome measure of the SCAT 2. The clinical usefulness of multiple components of the SCAT such as the SAC and BESS diminish in their sensitivity and specificity to SC 48 hours after injury, reinforcing its use as a screening tool after injury rather than to be used when making a return-to-play decision.[87,96,97] Additionally, health care professionals must be cognizant of the environment in which the SCAT is administered, because sideline administration has been demonstrated to influence performance on one or more components of the assessment.[98]

More recently, clinical measures based on visual tasks have been introduced as viable sideline measures of SC. Most notably, the King-Devick (K-D) test has gained attention as a promising sideline measure of SC. The K-D test is a rapid visual screening tool that assesses the speed and accuracy of an athlete reading numbers from left to right in increasingly complex patterns provided on alternative cards, which requires the use of saccades and concentration to complete.[99,100] Increasing time to completion on the K-D test is purported to reflect impaired eye movements, which is suggestive of suboptimal brain function.[93,100] The K-D test has been demonstrated to have strong evidence of test–retest reliability,[99–102] sensitivity, and specificity[103] with variable test–retest intervals across a wide range of age, sport, and nonsport groups.[104,105] Additionally, preliminary evidence suggests sex does not seem to influence K-D test performance.[106] Thus far, the evidence remains promising for the K-D test as a sideline measure of SC. Caution is warranted if using the K-D test beyond the acute period of injury because a dearth of literature exists addressing its long-term test–retest reliability, sensitivity, and specificity.

Symptom Report

Aside from being an interesting research finding, the fact that female athletes report more symptoms at both baseline and postinjury has very important implications for postinjury return-to-play management.[4,107–110] If the practitioner abides by the rule that an athlete should be asymptomatic before initiating a return-to-play protocol without awareness of the female's baseline symptom report, current symptoms could be interpreted as persistent difficulties when in fact, she may have experienced these symptoms before the injury. Researchers have also reported sex differences in terms of the quality of symptoms. Female athletes seem to report more somatic symptoms, cognitive functioning difficulties, emotional changes, and disrupted sleep compared with males.[41,111] The evidence pertaining to sex differences in recovery times is inconclusive, ranging from no sex differences to suggesting that female athletes take up to a 7 days longer than male athletes to be cleared to play. One consideration that may account for the discrepant findings is that the diagnosis of concussion and return-to-play decision is to some degree based on self-report symptom endorsement and females have been shown to be more honest and to volunteer information related to postconcussive symptoms more readily than males.[112] Practitioners managing female concussions should be aware of this variability in symptom endorsement and adapt their return-to-play and concussion management suggestions accordingly.[113]

Clinic-Based Assessment

If an athlete is removed from play owing to a suspected or diagnosed SC, a more extensive evaluation may take place in the clinic setting. Throughout the resolution of SC, the athlete should be evaluated systematically for concussion-related symptomology along with an assessment of cognitive and balance abilities. Since 1997, a multidimensional approach consisting of clinical measures of cognition, balance, and symptomology has been recommended for the management of SC to compliment the clinical examination.[48,54,114] A variety of clinical measures have been introduced to the marketplace to assist clinicians in diagnosing and managing SCs. In some cases, the marketing for some clinical measures has outpaced the data supporting their clinical usefulness.[115] A recent survey by Buckley and colleagues[116] reported that an increasing number of athletic trainers use the recommended multidimensional approach at baseline (41.9%), during the acute phase of injury (76.4%), and when making a return to play decision (63.9%) compared with previous reports.[117–119] In addition to the baseline assessment, the aforementioned clinical measures are typically readministered within 48 hours of injury, when the athlete reports symptom free, or at both time points.[116,117] The most commonly used clinical measures for primarily clinic-based acute and return-to-play assessments are many of the same measures used during baseline evaluations and include CNTs, clinical measures of balance, and self-reported symptoms.[116]

During the past 2 decades, CNTs have become a common component of SC policies at all levels of sport. The most commonly used CNT by surveyed athletic trainers (≥90%) is the ImPACT, with a minority of athletic trainers using CogState (Axon) or other platforms.[116,117,120] CNTs offer several advantages to traditional neuropsychological examinations, including a centralized means of data storage, ease and standardization of administration, and the availability of alternate forms to reduce practice effects.[68,115,121] Even so, 2 systematic reviews published in 2005 and 2013 indicated that, despite their routine use for the management of SC, several CNTs have been demonstrated to have suboptimal evidence of objectivity, reliability, and validity.[68,115] In terms of test–retest reliability, a recent study by Nelson and colleagues[122] compared the test–retest reliability of 3 CNTs (Automated Neuropsychological Assessment Metrics, Axon, and ImPACT) across several time points and reported reliability coefficients between 0.34 and 0.82 across platform outcomes scores. These findings are similar to another comparison study by Cole and colleagues[123] performed in military personnel. Nelson and colleagues[122] also compared the sensitivity of the 3 CNTs at 24 hours after injury, which ranged from 47.6% to 67.8%, and diminished at subsequent time points. These findings are similar to those of related studies.[124,125]

Sex has been reported to be a factor associated with CNT performance. A recent study investigated factors that influence baseline performance on ImPACT outcomes. Sex differences were reported for verbal and visual memory and reaction time outcomes scores, which is consistent with related literature.[108,126,127] These data support the need for sex-based normative values in absence of baseline data when making clinical decisions after an SC. Clinicians must be cognizant of several considerations when opting to use a CNT in their concussion policy. These considerations include training to properly administer and interpret CNT test results, ensure all hardware and software is not only up to date, but also standardized between computers, and providing a testing environment that will minimize distractions while completing a test before or after an SC.[78,80,82]

In terms of the clinic-based assessment of balance, the BESS has been reported routinely as the most common assessment of postural stability before and after concussion, followed by the Romberg test and the Sensory Organization Test (SOT).[116,117] Although used by surveyed athletic trainers, the Romberg test is a gross measure of postural stability and has little evidence to support its use in the clinical management of SC.[128] The SOT, a computerized measure of postural stability and the gold standard for balance assessment, however, it is prohibitive in terms of cost for most secondary school, collegiate and clinical settings.[129,130] The SOT consists of 18 trials that last 20 seconds. During each trial, athletes are instructed to maintain their balance during 6 sensory challenges designed to assess somatosensory, visual, and vestibular sensory inputs. As with CNTs, the SOT has been reported to have weak (0.35) to strong (0.93) test–retest reliability, sensitivity (12.8%–72.5%), and specificity (85.0%–94.9%).[124,125,131] There is limited to no evidence exists to show sex differences on any aforementioned clinical measure of balance.[4]

Historically, after an SC, physical rest has been prescribed until the athlete reports being symptom free.[95,132] Upon the athlete reporting symptom free, a stepwise graded exercise return to play has been recommended by several governing health care bodies. The purpose of the graded exercise protocol is to gradually increase an athlete's workload from light exercise to full-contact participation over approximately 5 days to determine the presence of lingering symptomology. Upon completion of sport-specific and noncontact drills, athletes are returned to play after an approved health care provider's clearance.[95] Since 2010, the concept of cognitive rest has emerged to supplement the traditional return-to-play protocol.

Anecdotally, as with physical activity, cognitive exertion (eg, looking at PowerPoints, reading textbooks) has been suggested to increase symptoms after an SC. Academic modification (eg, printing off PowerPoint slides, excused absences from school, homework extensions) along with more formalized plans such as an individualized education plan or a 504 plan have been recommended for the management of concussed student-athletes. Although similar, an individualized education plan and a 504 plan are different. Individualized education plans allows for specialized instruction, whereas a 504 plan allows for academic accommodations including services or changes in the environment to ensure a student with disabilities academic success. Although evidence-based protocols currently do not exist to guide clinical decision making in terms of progressively returning an athlete to the classroom, several theoretic papers and guidelines have been introduced to assist clinicians with the management of concussed student-athletes.[133–135] The majority of these reviews suggest an individualized rather than systematic approach to returning a student to the classroom after an SC, because each diagnosed injury will have a highly variable clinical presentation. Clinicians should evaluate each athlete's specific symptom phenotype to determine which academic modifications or formalized plans are appropriate to facilitate recovery. **Fig. 2** provides a theoretic timeline inclusive of both return-to-learn and return-to-play considerations.

PROLONGED RECOVERY FROM SPORT CONCUSSION
Risk Factors for a Protracted Recovery

One of the earliest studies to find sex differences in outcome after sports-related concussion examined 155 high school and college athletes who sustained concussions; 25% of participants were female.[41] Using an objective CNT and subjective symptom reports, female athletes experienced greater declines in cognitive performance and reported an increased symptom burden compared with male athletes. Given the large number of male athletes who participated in contact sports such as football and lacrosse, the authors speculated that helmets may have mitigated the consequences of SC related to concussion-related symptomology and cognitive deficits. However, a comparison between female athletes (none of whom had helmets) and male athletes with and without helmets yielded the same results. Even after controlling for the potential protective effects of helmets, female athletes had more objective and subjective symptoms of SC despite being evaluated an average of 24 hours after than male athletes. In a separate study of soccer players, females reported more symptoms and demonstrated slower reaction time on a CNT after concussion.[60] Other researchers found that young female athletes (ages 9–17) took longer than males to

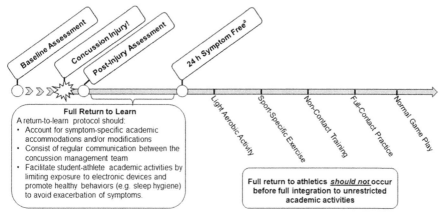

Fig. 2. A general overview of the return to play timeline after a concussion. The postinjury assessments may provide athlete-specific information relative to impairment, including symptomology. This information can be used to guide re-integration into activities of daily living, especially as they relate to the return to learning. The return to play progression as put forth by the most recent Concussion in Sport Group[48] should not occur before the athlete has reported symptom free and also not before the athlete has completed a return to learn progression. [a] Typically 7 to 10 days after injury.

become symptom free.[136] A separate study reported that sex differences disappeared when controlling for baseline differences in symptom reporting.[137] An extensive review of the literature on sex differences in recovery from sports concussion conducted by the International Consensus Conference on Concussion in Sport Group[138] found mixed results with equal numbers of studies supporting or disproving differences in outcome. There was some evidence that young women and girls have an increased risk for concussions symptoms lasting longer than a month.

Preexisting Mood Disorder

Much of what we have learned about recovery from sports concussion is based on studies conducted on individuals who have sustained mTBI from mechanisms of injury outside of sport. One such study found intriguing predictors of a longer, more complicated recovery after mTBI.[139] Participants consisted of emergency department patients who were admitted shortly after injury and those who had orthopedic injuries, but not mTBI. The strongest predictors of postconcussion symptoms 1 week after injury included the diagnosis of a concussion, female sex, a premorbid psychiatric history, and anxiety symptoms at the time of follow-up. Three months after injury, the strongest predictor of postconcussion symptoms was preinjury physical or psychiatric history. Anxiety was a significant predictor of continued symptoms at 3 months in those who had the mTBI, and posttraumatic and/or general life stress was also predictive of endorsed postconcussion symptoms at this time point in the orthopedic injury group. This prospective study was important in highlighting that preexisting and postconcussion psychiatric symptoms, especially anxiety, predicted long-term postconcussion symptoms. Other researchers found that depression, anxiety, and "neuroticism" in patients who experienced either mTBI, spinal cord injury, or no injury were stronger predictors of postconcussion symptoms than neuropsychological test results, although the latter did predict cognitive symptoms in the group with mTBI.[140]

Similarly, a study of Division I collegiate athletes found that baseline depression was the most significant predictor of depression and anxiety after SC.[141]

In a systematic review of multivariate models of mTBI, the most robust predictors were preinjury mental health, acute postinjury anxiety, and neuropsychological results shortly after mTBI.[142] In addition, females had worse outcomes. Notably, the severity of the mTBI had little predictive value. A prospective study of biopsychosocial factors affecting outcome after mTBI found that significant predictors of symptoms 1 month after injury were preinjury mental health and peripheral injury and depression at the time of follow-up.[143] The authors summarized that postconcussion symptomology is complex, unique to each individual, and likely reflects multiple factors, including preexisting mental health, current life stress, depression, personality factors, chronic pain, genetics, and potentially other environmental and psychosocial factors. They conclude by commenting that "the extent to which damage to the structure of the brain contributes to the persistence of PCS remains unclear."[143]

Clinical Assessment of Protracted Recovery

For athletes who experience prolonged recoveries after a concussion, specialty evaluation and care can be critical in identifying specific factors that may be impeding recovery. In particular, multidisciplinary care has been identified as important in providing consistent care and reducing health care use.[144] Based on an extensive review of empirical literature, updated clinical practice guidelines for the management of concussion were identified by a group in Ontario.[17] The Ontario group recommended that any individual with persisting concussion symptoms receive a thorough evaluation of physical, cognitive, behavioral, and emotional symptoms and they remind providers that persisting symptoms are likely owing to multiple factors. Factors contributing to prolonged recovery after concussion can include posttraumatic headaches, disruption of the sleep–wake cycle, mental health concerns, persisting cognitive symptoms including but not limited to premorbid attention deficit hyperactivity disorder or learning disorders, visual dysfunction, persisting dizziness or difficulty with balance, and prolonged fatigue. The Ontario guidelines provide extensive recommendations for the evaluation and treatment of each of these factors.[17]

Headaches after concussion are the most common symptom and can often persist.[145] Given that concussed athletes who display migraine headache symptoms take longer to recover after injury, the existence of this symptom has been speculated to translate to a longer recovery time for female athletes.[113,146,147] A variety of pharmacologic treatments are available starting with over the counter medications and progressing to prophylactic medication and abortive medications, particularly for those who develop migraine-type headaches.[17] In addition to medication, nonpharmacologic treatments such as massage, relaxation techniques, cognitive–behavioral therapy, and acupressure or acupuncture may be helpful in reducing headache pain. Those athletes with persisting headaches should also be evaluated for visual dysfunction because the latter can trigger headaches, particularly when using electronic devices or completing reading assignments.

Deficits in visual function can occur after concussion and affect recovery. Common visual difficulties after concussion include photosensitivity and convergence insufficiency, as well as disruption of saccades and antisaccades, smooth pursuit, accommodation, and the vestibular–ocular reflex.[148] Some of the visual difficulties are associated with cognitive deficits such as attention dysfunction that can affect visual tracking. In a study of adolescents, 69% had some form of visual dysfunction after concussion with approximately one-half demonstrating accommodation insufficiency or convergence insufficiency.[149] In a review of postconcussion visual symptoms, Heinmiller and Gunton[150] reported evidence that patients who present with vestibuloocular dysfunction have a 4-fold increased risk of postconcussion syndrome. The Convergence Insufficiency Symptom Survey—Revised (Rouse and colleagues 2004) is a validated 15-item checklist that can be used as a screening measure of vestibuloocular dysfunction and is also used an outcome measure to track recovery and response to treatment, although some have presented evidence that elevated scores are not specific to convergence insufficiency and scores may vary depending on whether it is administered by a practitioner or self-administered by the patient.[151,152]

Patients with convergence insufficiency after concussion may be prescribed a variety of therapies, including formal clinic-based vision therapy and home-based exercises such as "pencil pushups." For pencil pushups, patients are asked to focus on the tip of a pencil held at arm's length. The pencil is then moved toward the patient's nose until diplopia is expressed and then the pencil is moved back to arm's length. Pencil pushups may be prescribed several times a week to treat convergence insufficiency. A randomized clinical trial of these treatments in young adults that compared in-clinic vision therapy, an in-clinic vision therapy placebo or home-based pencil pushups, found that all 3 groups demonstrated significantly reduced symptoms.[153] Those receiving an in-clinic treatment or placebo demonstrated greater improvement than those assigned to home exercises and more than one-half the participants were improved, but still symptomatic after treatment.

Vestibular dysfunction after an SC can also contribute to prolonged recovery and an extensive review of common postconcussion vestibular disorders may be found elsewhere.[154] Benign paroxysmal positional vertigo can occur after a concussion owing to the dislodging of otoconia, which are colloquially referred to as "crystals in the ear" into the semicircular canals, resulting in vertigo consequential of head movement. The Dix-Hallpike Maneuver followed by a canalith repositioning maneuver is the recommended intervention for those with otoconia.[17] Postconcussion deficits in balance or postural control may be related to disruption of sensory integration and should be evaluated further by a specialist in vestibular rehabilitation.[17,154] Balance deficits after SC were also found to be associated with posttraumatic headaches, possibly owing to increased difficulty with sensory organization.[155]

Persisting dizziness may be related to vestibular dysfunction or may reflect cervicogenic dizziness, both of which require further evaluation and treatment by a specialist.[154] Vestibular rehabilitation therapy (VRT) is often recommended for those with postconcussion balance impairment, dizziness, or vertigo. In a systematic review of published outcome studies of VRT, only 10 studies met the inclusion criteria.[154] The included studies evaluated a variety of interventions including VRT combined with multimodal interventions consisting of strength training, manual therapy, occupational tasks, counseling/education, or medication. Although there was no level 1 evidence to support that VRT improved dizziness, balance, or gait impairment, there was level 1 evidence supporting that participation in VRT is beneficial in earlier return to sport after concussion.

Although some athletics programs have clinical neuropsychologists actively involved in the preseason baseline assessment process as well as diagnosis and management of sports concussions, other programs have limited access to neuropsychologists and only refer athletes with persisting symptoms.[116] Athletes should be referred for formal neuropsychological evaluation when there is concern about declining cognitive function after an SC.[156] Concerns about the cumulative effects of multiple SCs and consideration of retirement also warrant referral.[156] A neuropsychological evaluation is recommended when:

- Postconcussion symptoms persist longer than expected (2 weeks for adult athletes);
- The athlete has a history of multiple concussions, the presence of postconcussion seizures, or positive neuroimaging findings;
- The athlete has a premorbid history of attention deficit hyperactivity disorder, learning disorder, migraines, and/or seizures; and/or
- The athlete seems to have a psychological reaction to their injury and/or a significant premorbid history of depression or anxiety that may be complicating recovery, and/or the need for academic accommodations.

Neuropsychological evaluation of athletes with attention deficit hyperactivity disorder or learning disorders is often necessary because the premorbid attention deficits or learning disorder symptoms can complicate interpretation of CNT performance after an SC. A comprehensive neuropsychological evaluation consists of a clinical interview assessing cognitive symptoms, mood evaluation, medical and psychological history, and evaluation of psychosocial factors that may be contributing to persisting symptoms. A variety of cognitive functions are evaluated, including but not limited to attention, processing speed, verbal and visual learning and memory, and problem solving, through individually administered paper and pencil tests. Tests of performance validity and personality testing are administered typically to evaluate for nonneurologic factors that may be contributing to the prolonged symptom course. The mood assessment and psychological history can often identify premorbid or concurrent psychological factors associated with a prolonged recovery after SC.[157] Even in athletes with minimal to no significant medical or psychological history, preconcussion somatization has been associated with postconcussion symptom duration and somatic concerns can be identified during the neuropsychological evaluation.[158]

For those athletes with persisting cognitive symptoms, the neuropsychologist can suggest compensatory strategies and recommend academic accommodations (if not already in place). Neuropsychologists may uncover additional postconcussion symptoms, such as headaches, sleep disturbance, or visual or vestibular dysfunction, that may be contributing to cognitive symptoms and should work with the multidisciplinary treatment team (eg, physicians and athletic trainers) to ensure that referral to other specialists are made. Athletes with significant psychological factors should be provided education about the role of anxiety, depression, and other mood symptoms in prolonging recovery and referred to a sports psychologist, clinical psychologist, or other mental health provider for treatment.[159] Concerns regarding suboptimal effort on neuropsychological tests should be discussed with the athlete as he or she may have concerns about returning to sport owing to concerns about the potential cumulative effects of concussions. Discussions and concerns about retirement from sport may arise through the process of neuropsychological evaluation and can provide a valuable clinical service to the athlete and the treatment team.

RECOMMENDATIONS FOR THE MANAGEMENT OF FEMALE ATHLETES WITH SPORT CONCUSSION

The purpose of the current review was to address sex-related differences which may influence the management of SC. During the past 20 years, myriad investigations have sought to examine the differences between male and female athletes in terms of preinjury and postinjury considerations. Despite evidence of sex differences in terms of neuropsychological test performance, symptom reporting and neck strength differences, other preliminary differences in terms of concussion preliminary findings have been refuted with more recent investigations. Overall, clinical recommendations for the management of the concussed female athlete include the following.

- Establishing preinjury symptom burden and psychological history. Females tend to report a higher symptom burden during their baseline assessments compared with males. Clinicians should record and refer to baseline symptom reports when making clinical decisions after an SC.
- Preliminary evidence of physical and physiologic differences such as neck strength and hormone levels (ie, progesterone) suggest female athletes are potentially predisposed to sustaining SCs and experiencing prolonged recoveries.
- Return to play should only occur after a successful integration into unrestricted academic activities.
- Although some studies have reported sex differences in terms of duration of recovery and performance on clinical measures, the data remain equivocal, which reinforces the need for an individualized approach for concussion management, regardless of biological sex.

SUMMARY

The purpose of the current review was to summarize the ever-growing body of literature surrounding SC and the female athlete. The current literature supports sex differences on preinjury and postinjury neurocognitive test performance, symptom reporting, and susceptibility to and potential risk for protracted recoveries from SC. Taking this evidence into account, the authors support the need for an individualized approach to SC management based on premorbid functioning, individual risk factors, and clinical presentation after injury, regardless of biological sex.

REFERENCES

1. Fedor A, Gunstad J. Would you let your child play football? Attitudes toward football safety. Appl Neuropsychol Child 2016;5(2):107–9.
2. Powell JW, Barber-Foss KD. Traumatic brain injury in high school athletes. JAMA 1999;282(10):958–63.
3. Covassin T, Moran R, Elbin RJ. Sex differences in reported concussion injury rates and time loss from participation: an update of the National Collegiate Athletic Association Injury Surveillance Program from 2004-2005 through 2008-2009. J Athl Train 2016;51(3):189–94.
4. Covassin T, Elbin RJ, Harris W, et al. The role of age and sex in symptoms, neurocognitive performance, and postural stability in athletes after concussion. Am J Sports Med 2012;40(6):1303–12. Available at: http://ajs.sagepub.com/content/40/6/1303.full.pdf.
5. Sandel NK, Schatz P, Goldberg KB, et al. Sex-based differences in cognitive deficits and symptom reporting among acutely concussed adolescent lacrosse and soccer players. Am J Sports Med 2016;45(4):937–44.
6. Marar M, McIlvain NM, Fields SK, et al. Epidemiology of concussions among United States high school athletes in 20 sports. Am J Sports Med 2012;40(4):747–55.
7. Lincoln AE, Caswell SV, Almquist JL, et al. Trends in concussion incidence in high school sports: a prospective 11-year study. Am J Sports Med 2011;39(5):958–63.

8. Zuckerman SL, Kerr ZY, Yengo-Kahn A, et al. Epidemiology of sports-related concussion in NCAA athletes from 2009-2010 to 2013-2014: incidence, recurrence, and mechanisms. Am J Sports Med 2015;43(11):2654–62.

9. Gessel LM, Fields SK, Collins CL, et al. Concussions among United States high school and collegiate athletes. J Athl Train 2007;42(4):495–503.

10. Castile L, Collins CL, McIlvain NM, et al. The epidemiology of new versus recurrent sports concussions among high school athletes, 2005-2010. Br J Sports Med 2012;46(8):603–10.

11. Covassin T, Swanik CB, Sachs ML. Epidemiological considerations of concussions among intercollegiate athletes. Appl Neuropsychol 2003;10(1):12–22.

12. Dompier TP, Kerr ZY, Marshall SW, et al. Incidence of concussion during practice and games in youth, high school, and collegiate American football players. JAMA Pediatr 2015;169(7):659–65.

13. Kerr ZY, Roos KG, Djoko A, et al. Epidemiologic measures for quantifying the incidence of concussion in National Collegiate Athletic Association Sports. J Athl Train 2016;52(3):167–74.

14. Khodaee M, Currie DW, Asif IM, et al. Nine-year study of US high school soccer injuries: data from a national sports injury surveillance programme. Br J Sports Med 2016;51:185–93.

15. King H, Campbell S, Herzog M, et al. Epidemiology of injuries in high school football: does school size matter? J Phys Act Health 2015;12(8):1162–7.

16. Lincoln AE, Hinton RY, Almquist JL, et al. Head, face, and eye injuries in scholastic and collegiate lacrosse: a 4-year prospective study. Am J Sports Med 2007;35(2):207–15.

17. Marshall S, Bayley M, McCullagh S, et al. Updated clinical practice guidelines for concussion/mild traumatic brain injury and persistent symptoms. Brain Inj 2015;29(6):688–700.

18. Reeser JC, Gregory A, Berg RL, et al. A comparison of women's collegiate and girls' high school volleyball injury data collected prospectively over a 4-year period. Sports Health 2015;7(6):504–10.

19. Roos KG, Wasserman EB, Dalton SL, et al. Epidemiology of 3825 injuries sustained in six seasons of National Collegiate Athletic Association men's and women's soccer (2009/2010-2014/2015). Br J Sports Med 2017;51(13):1029–34.

20. Rosenthal JA, Foraker RE, Collins CL, et al. National high school athlete concussion rates from 2005-2006 to 2011-2012. Am J Sports Med 2014;42(7):1710–5.

21. Shankar PR, Fields SK, Collins CL, et al. Epidemiology of high school and collegiate football injuries in the United States, 2005-2006. Am J Sports Med 2007;35(8):1295–303.

22. Yard EE, Collins CL, Dick RW, et al. An epidemiologic comparison of high school and college wrestling injuries. Am J Sports Med 2008;36(1):57–64.

23. Boden BP, Kirkendall DT, Garrett WE Jr. Concussion incidence in elite college soccer players. Am J Sports Med 1998;26(2):238–41.

24. Tierney RT, Sitler MR, Swanik CB, et al. Gender differences in head-neck segment dynamic stabilization during head acceleration. Med Sci Sports Exerc 2005;37(2):272–9.

25. Gutierrez GM, Conte C, Lightbourne K. The relationship between impact force, neck strength, and neurocognitive performance in soccer heading in adolescent females. Pediatr Exerc Sci 2014;26(1):33–40.

26. Bretzin AC, Mansell JL, Tierney RT, et al. Sex differences in anthropometrics and heading kinematics among division I soccer athletes. Sports Health 2017;9(2): 168–73.

27. Tierney RT, Higgins M, Caswell SV, et al. Sex differences in head acceleration during heading while wearing soccer headgear. J Athl Train 2008;43(6):578–84.

28. Collins CL, Fletcher EN, Fields SK, et al. Neck strength: a protective factor reducing risk for concussion in high school sports. J Prim Prev 2014;35(5): 309–19.

29. Kelly DF, Gonzalo IT, Cohan P, et al. Hypopituitarism following traumatic brain injury and aneurysmal subarachnoid hemorrhage: a preliminary report. J Neurosurg 2000;93(5):743–52.

30. Benvenga S, Campenni A, Ruggeri RM, et al. Clinical review 113: hypopituitarism secondary to head trauma. J Clin Endocrinol Metab 2000;85(4):1353–61.

31. Klose M, Juul A, Struck J, et al. Acute and long-term pituitary insufficiency in traumatic brain injury: a prospective single-centre study. Clin Endocrinol (Oxf) 2007;67(4):598–606.

32. Popovic V, Aimaretti G, Casanueva FF, et al. Hypopituitarism following traumatic brain injury. Growth Horm IGF Res 2005;15(3):177–84.

33. Schneider M, Schneider HJ, Yassouridis A, et al. Predictors of anterior pituitary insufficiency after traumatic brain injury. Clin Endocrinol (Oxf) 2008;68(2): 206–12.

34. Tanriverdi F, Kelestimur F. Pituitary dysfunction following traumatic brain injury: clinical perspectives. Neuropsychiatr Dis Treat 2015;11:1835–43.

35. Agha A, Phillips J, Thompson CJ. Hypopituitarism following traumatic brain injury (TBI). Br J Neurosurg 2007;21(2):210–6.

36. Norman AW, Litwack G. Hormones. 2nd edition. New York: Academic Press; 1997.

37. Bazarian JJ, Blyth B, Mookerjee S, et al. Sex differences in outcome after mild traumatic brain injury. J Neurotrauma 2010;27(3):527–39.

38. Viano DC, Lovsund P. Biomechanics of brain and spinal cord injury: analysis of neuropathologic and neurophysiologic experiments. J Crash Prev Inj Control 1999;1(1):35–43.

39. Viano DC, Casson IR, Pellman EJ, et al. Concussion in professional football: brain responses by finite element analysis: part 9. Neurosurgery 2005;57(5): 891–916 [discussion: 891–916].

40. Wang Y, Nelson LD, LaRoche AA, et al. Cerebral blood flow alterations in acute sport-related concussion. J Neurotrauma 2016;33(13):1227–36.

41. Broshek DK, Kaushik T, Freeman JR, et al. Sex differences in outcome following sports-related concussion. J Neurosurg 2005;102(5):856–63.

42. Wunderle K, Hoeger KM, Wasserman E, et al. Menstrual phase as predictor of outcome after mild traumatic brain injury in women. J Head Trauma Rehabil 2014;29(5):E1–8.

43. Moller-Nielsen J, Hammar M. Women's soccer injuries in relation to the menstrual cycle and oral contraceptive use. Med Sci Sports Exerc 1989;21(2): 126–9.

44. Decloe MD, Meeuwisse WH, Hagel BE, et al. Injury rates, types, mechanisms and risk factors in female youth ice hockey. Br J Sports Med 2014;48(1):51–6.

45. Giza CC, Kutcher JS, Ashwal S, et al. Summary of evidence-based guideline update: evaluation and management of concussion in sports: report of the Guideline Development Subcommittee of the American Academy of Neurology. Neurology 2013;80(24):2250–7.

46. Harmon KG, Drezner J, Gammons M, et al. American medical society for sports medicine position statement: concussion in sport. Clin J Sport Med 2013;23(1): 1–18.

47. Halstead ME, Walter KD. Clinical sport-related concussion in children and adolescents. Pediatrics 2010;126(3):597–615.

48. McCrory P, Meeuwisse WH, Aubry M, et al. Consensus statement on concussion in sport-the 4th International Conference on Concussion in Sport held in Zurich, November 2012. PM R 2013;5(4):255–79.

49. Chamard E, Lassonde M, Henry L, et al. Neurometabolic and microstructural alterations following a sports-related concussion in female athletes. Brain Inj 2013; 27(9):1038–46.

50. Bazarian JJ, Zhu T, Blyth B, et al. Subject-specific changes in brain white matter on diffusion tensor imaging after sports-related concussion. Magn Reson Imaging 2012;30(2):171–80.

51. Lancaster MA, Olson DV, McCrea MA, et al. Acute white matter changes following sport-related concussion: a serial diffusion tensor and diffusion kurtosis tensor imaging study. Hum Brain Mapp 2016;37(11):3821–34.

52. Cubon VA, Putukian M, Boyer C, et al. A diffusion tensor imaging study on the white matter skeleton in individuals with sports-related concussion. J Neurotrauma 2011;28(2):189–201.

53. Chamard E, Lefebvre G, Lassonde M, et al. Long-term abnormalities in the corpus callosum of female concussed athletes. J Neurotrauma 2016;33(13): 1220–6.

54. Broglio SP, Cantu RC, Gioia GA, et al, National Athletic Trainer's Association. National Athletic Trainers' Association position statement: management of sport concussion. J Athl Train 2014;49(2):245–65.

55. Schmidt JD, Register-Mihalik JK, Mihalik JP, et al. Identifying impairments after concussion: normative data versus individualized baselines. Med Sci Sports Exerc 2012;44(9):1621–8.

56. Randolph C. Baseline neuropsychological testing in managing sport-related concussion: does it modify risk? Curr Sports Med Rep 2011;10(1):21–6.

57. Collins MW, Grindel SH, Lovell MR, et al. Relationship between concussion and neuropsychological performance in college football players. JAMA 1999; 282(10):964–70.

58. Kontos AP, Covassin T, Elbin RJ, et al. Depression and neurocognitive performance after concussion among male and female high school and collegiate athletes. Arch Phys Med Rehabil 2012;93(10):1751–6.

59. Collins MW, Lovell MR, Iverson GL, et al. Cumulative effects of concussion in high school athletes. Neurosurgery 2002;51(5):1175–9 [discussion: 1180–1].

60. Colvin AC, Mullen J, Lovell MR, et al. The role of concussion history and gender in recovery from soccer-related concussion. Am J Sports Med 2009;37(9): 1699–704.

61. Iverson GL, Brooks BL, Lovell MR, et al. No cumulative effects for one or two previous concussions. Br J Sports Med 2006;40(1):72–5.

62. Martini DN, Sabin MJ, DePesa SA, et al. The chronic effects of concussion on gait. Arch Phys Med Rehabil 2011;92(4):585–9.

63. Sosnoff JJ, Broglio SP, Shin S, et al. Previous mild traumatic brain injury and postural-control dynamics. J Athletic Train 2011;46(1):85–91.

64. Iverson GL, Gaetz M, Lovell MR, et al. Cumulative effects of concussion in amateur athletes. Brain Inj 2004;18(5):433–43.

65. Lovell MR, Collins MW. Neuropsychological assessment of the college football player. J Head Trauma Rehabil 1998;13(2):9–26.
66. Macciocchi SN, Barth JT, Alves W, et al. Neurological functioning and recovery after mild head injury in collegiate athletes. Neurosurgery 1996;39:510–4.
67. Grindel SH, Lovell MR, Collins MW. The assessment of sport-related concussion: the evidence behind neuropsychological testing and management. Clin J Sport Med 2001;11(3):134–43.
68. Randolph C, McCrea M, Barr WB. Is neuropsychological testing useful in the management of sport-related concussion? J Athl Train 2005;40(3):139–52.
69. Echemendia RJ, Julian LJ. Mild traumatic brain injury in sports: neuropsychology's contribution to a developing field. Neuropsychol Rev 2001;11(2):69–88.
70. Brandt J. The Hopkins verbal learning test: development of a new memory test with six equivalent forms. Clin Neuropsychol 1991;2:125–42.
71. Smith A. Symbol digit modalities test (SDMT) manual. Revised edition. Los Angeles (CA): Western Psychological Services; 1982.
72. Reitan RM. Validity of the trail-making test as an indicator in organic brain damage. Percept Mot Skills 1958;8:271–6.
73. Spreen O, Strauss E. A compendium of neuropsychological tests. 3rd edition. New York: Oxford University Press; 2006.
74. Wechlser D. Wechsler adult intelligence scale (WAIS-III) manual. New York: Psychological Corporation; 1997.
75. Trenerry MR, Crosson B, DeBoe J, et al. Stroop: neuropsychological screening test. Odessa (FL): Psychological Assessment Resources; 1989.
76. Cegalis JA. Software for testing concentration and attention manual. Nashua (NH): Forthought Ltd; 1991.
77. Bauer RM, Iverson GL, Cernich AN, et al. Computerized neuropsychological assessment devices: joint position paper of the American Academy of Clinical Neuropsychology and the National Academy of Neuropsychology. Clin Neuropsychol 2012;26(2):177–96.
78. Moser RS, Schatz P, Neidzwski K, et al. Group versus individual administration affects baseline neurocognitive test performance. Am J Sports Med 2011; 39(11):2325–30.
79. Echemendia RJ, Iverson GL, McCrea M, et al. Advances in neuropsychological assessment of sport-related concussion. Br J Sports Med 2013;47(5):294–8.
80. Schatz P, Neidzwski K, Moser RS, et al. Relationship between subjective test feedback provided by high-school athletes during computer-based assessment of baseline cognitive functioning and self-reported symptoms. Arch Clin Neuropsychol 2010;25(4):285–92.
81. Covassin T, Elbin RJ 3rd, Stiller-Ostrowski JL, et al. Immediate post-concussion assessment and cognitive testing (ImPACT) practices of sports medicine professionals. J Athl Train 2009;44(6):639–44.
82. Rahman-Filipiak AA, Woodard JL. Administration and environment considerations in computer-based sports-concussion assessment. Neuropsychol Rev 2013;23(4):314–34.
83. Schatz P, Glatts C. "Sandbagging" baseline test performance on ImPACT, without detection, is more difficult than it appears. Arch Clin Neuropsychol 2013;28(3):236–44.
84. Erdal K. Neuropsychological testing for sports-related concussion: how athletes can sandbag their baseline testing without detection. Arch Clin Neuropsychol 2012;27(5):473–9.

85. Arnett P, Meyer J, Merritt V, et al. Neuropsychological testing in mild traumatic brain injury: what to do when baseline testing is not available. Sports Med Arthrosc 2016;24(3):116–22.

86. McCrea M, Kelly JP, Kluge J, et al. Standardized assessment of concussion in football players. Neurology 1997;48(3):586–8.

87. McCrea M. Standardized mental status testing on the sideline after sport-related concussion. J Athl Train 2001;36(3):274–9.

88. Valovich McLeod TC, Barr WB, McCrea M, et al. Psychometric and measurement properties of concussion assessment tools in youth sports. J Athl Train 2006;41(4):399–408.

89. Putukian M, Echemendia R, Dettwiler-Danspeckgruber A, et al. Prospective clinical assessment using Sideline Concussion Assessment Tool-2 testing in the evaluation of sport-related concussion in college athletes. Clin J Sport Med 2015;25(1):36–42.

90. Guskiewicz KM, Riemann BL, Perrin DH, et al. Alternative approaches to the assessment of mild head injury in athletes. Med Sci Sports Exerc 1997;29(7 Suppl):S213–21.

91. Finnoff JT, Peterson VJ, Hollman JH, et al. Intrarater and interrater reliability of the balance error scoring system (BESS). PM R 2009;1(1):50–4.

92. Bell DR, Guskiewicz KM, Clark MA, et al. Systematic review of the balance error scoring system. Sports Health 2011;3(3):287–95.

93. Resch JE, Kutcher JS. The acute management of sport concussion in pediatric athletes. J Child Neurol 2015;30(12):1686–94.

94. McCrory P, Johnston K, Meeuwisse W, et al. Summary and agreement statement of the 2nd International Conference on concussion in sport, Prague 2004. Br J Sports Med 2005;39(4):196–204.

95. McCrory P, Meeuwisse WH, Aubry M, et al. Consensus statement on concussion in sport: the 4(th) International Conference on concussion in sport held in Zurich, November 2012. J Am Coll Surg 2013;216(5):e55–71.

96. Riemann BL, Guskiewicz KM. Effects of mild head injury on postural stability as measured through clinical balance testing. J Athl Train 2000;35(1):19–25.

97. Valovich TC, Perrin DH, Gansneder BM. Repeat administration elicits a practice effect with the balance error scoring system but not with the standardized assessment of concussion in high school athletes. J Athl Train 2003;38(1):51–6.

98. Rahn C, Munkasy BA, Joyner AB, et al. Sideline performance of the balance error scoring system during a live sporting event. Clin J Sport Med 2015;25(3):248–53.

99. Alsalaheen B, Haines J, Yorke A, et al. King-Devick test reference values and associations with balance measures in high school American football players. Scand J Med Sci Sports 2016;26(2):235–9.

100. Galetta KM, Barrett J, Allen M, et al. The King-Devick test as a determinant of head trauma and concussion in boxers and MMA fighters. Neurology 2011;76(17):1456–62.

101. Galetta KM, Brandes LE, Maki K, et al. The King-Devick test and sports-related concussion: study of a rapid visual screening tool in a collegiate cohort. J Neurol Sci 2011;309(1–2):34–9.

102. King D, Hume P, Gissane C, et al. Use of the King-Devick test for sideline concussion screening in junior rugby league. J Neurol Sci 2015;357(1–2):75–9.

103. Leong DF, Balcer LJ, Galetta SL, et al. The King-Devick test for sideline concussion screening in collegiate football. J Optom 2015;8(2):131–9.

104. Walsh DV, Capo-Aponte JE, Beltran T, et al. Assessment of the King-Devick(R) (KD) test for screening acute mTBI/concussion in warfighters. J Neurol Sci 2016; 370:305–9.
105. Silverberg ND, Luoto TM, Ohman J, et al. Assessment of mild traumatic brain injury with the King-Devick Test® in an emergency department sample. Brain Inj 2014;28(12):1590–3.
106. Benedict PA, Baner NV, Harrold GK, et al. Gender and age predict outcomes of cognitive, balance and vision testing in a multidisciplinary concussion center. J Neurol Sci 2015;353(1–2):111–5.
107. Mihalik JP, Ondrak KS, Guskiewicz KM, et al. The effects of menstrual cycle phase on clinical measures of concussion in healthy college-aged females. J Sci Med Sport 2009;12(3):383–7.
108. Covassin T, Elbin RJ 3rd, Larson E, et al. Sex and age differences in depression and baseline sport-related concussion neurocognitive performance and symptoms. Clin J Sport Med 2012;22(2):98–104.
109. Sandel NK, Lovell MR, Kegel NE, et al. The relationship of symptoms and neurocognitive performance to perceived recovery from sports-related concussion among adolescent athletes. Appl Neuropsychol Child 2013;2(1):64–9.
110. Zuckerman SL, Apple RP, Odom MJ, et al. Effect of sex on symptoms and return to baseline in sport-related concussion. J Neurosurg Pediatr 2014;13(1):72–81.
111. Covassin T, Schatz P, Swanik CB. Sex differences in neuropsychological function and post-concussion symptoms of concussed collegiate athletes. Neurosurgery 2007;61(2):345–50 [discussion: 350–1].
112. Cantu RC, Guskiewicz K, Register-Mihalik JK. A retrospective clinical analysis of moderate to severe athletic concussions. PM R 2010;2(12):1088–93.
113. Covassin T, Elbin RJ. The female athlete: the role of gender in the assessment and management of sport-related concussion. Clin Sports Med 2011;30(1): 125–31, x.
114. Kelly JP, Rosenberg JH. Diagnosis and management of concussion in sports. Neurology 1997;48(3):575–80.
115. Resch JE, McCrea MA, Cullum CM. Computerized neurocognitive testing in the management of sport-related concussion: an update. Neuropsychol Rev 2013; 23(4):335–49.
116. Buckley TA, Burdette G, Kelly K. Concussion-management practice patterns of National Collegiate Athletic Association division II and III athletic trainers: how the other half lives. J Athl Train 2015;50(8):879–88.
117. Lynall RC, Laudner KG, Mihalik JP, et al. Concussion-assessment and -management techniques used by athletic trainers. J Athl Train 2013;48(6):844–50.
118. Notebaert AJ, Guskiewicz KM. Current trends in athletic training practice for concussion assessment and management. J Athl Train 2005;40(4):320–5.
119. Ferrara MS, McCrea M, Peterson CL, et al. A survey of practice patterns in concussion assessment and management. J Athl Train 2001;36(2):145–9.
120. Meehan WP 3rd, d'Hemecourt P, Collins CL, et al. Computerized neurocognitive testing for the management of sport-related concussions. Pediatrics 2012; 129(1):38–44.
121. Collie A, Maruff P. Computerised neuropsychological testing. Br J Sports Med 2003;37(1):2–3.
122. Nelson LD, LaRoche AA, Pfaller AY, et al. Prospective, head-to-head study of three computerized neurocognitive assessment tools (CNTs): reliability and validity for the assessment of sport-related concussion. J Int Neuropsychol Soc 2016;22(1):24–37.

123. Cole WR, Arrieux JP, Schwab K, et al. Test-retest reliability of four computerized neurocognitive assessment tools in an active duty military population. Arch Clin Neuropsychol 2013;28(7):732–42.

124. Broglio SP, Macciocchi SN, Ferrara MS. Sensitivity of the concussion assessment battery. Neurosurgery 2007;60(6):1050–7 [discussion: 1057–8].

125. Resch JE, Brown CN, Schmidt J, et al. The sensitivity and specificity of clinical measures of sport concussion: three tests are better than one. BMJ Open Sport Exerc Med 2016;2(e000012):1–10.

126. Hall E, Cottle J, Ketcham C, et al. Concussion baseline testing: preexisting factors, symptoms, and neurocognitive performance. J Athl Train 2017;52(2): 77–81.

127. Brown CN, Guskiewicz KM, Bleiberg J. Athlete characteristics and outcome scores for computerized neuropsychological assessment: a preliminary analysis. J Athletic Train 2007;42(4):515–23.

128. Murray N, Salvatore A, Powell D, et al. Reliability and validity evidence of multiple balance assessments in athletes with a concussion. J Athl Train 2014;49(4):540–9.

129. Guskiewicz KM. Balance assessment in the management of sport-related concussion. Clin Sports Med 2011;30(1):89–102, ix.

130. Guskiewicz KM. Postural stability assessment following concussion: one piece of the puzzle. Clin J Sport Med 2001;11(3):182–9.

131. Register-Mihalik JK, Guskiewicz KM, Mihalik JP, et al. Reliable change, sensitivity, and specificity of a multidimensional concussion assessment battery: implications for caution in clinical practice. J head Trauma Rehabil 2012; 28(4):274–83.

132. Aubry M, Cantu R, Dvorak J, et al. Summary and agreement statement of the 1st international symposium on concussion in sport, Vienna 2001. Clin J Sport Med 2002;12(1):6–11.

133. Master CL, Gioia GA, Leddy JJ, et al. Importance of 'return-to-learn' in pediatric and adolescent concussion. Pediatr Ann 2012;41(9):1–6.

134. DeMatteo C, Stazyk K, Giglia L, et al. A balanced protocol for return to school for children and youth following concussive injury. Clin Pediatr (Phila) 2015;54(8): 783–92.

135. Halstead ME, McAvoy K, Devore CD, et al. Returning to learning following a concussion. Pediatrics 2013;132(5):948–57.

136. Berz K, Divine J, Foss KB, et al. Sex-specific differences in the severity of symptoms and recovery rate following sports-related concussion in young athletes. Phys Sportsmed 2013;41(2):58–63.

137. Baker JG, Leddy JJ, Darling SR, et al. Gender differences in recovery from sports-related concussion in adolescents. Clin Pediatr (Phila) 2016;55(8):771–5.

138. Conference Proceedings. Paper presented at: International Consensus Conference on Concussion in Sport October 27–28, 2016. Berlin (GA), 2016.

139. Ponsford J, Cameron P, Fitzgerald M, et al. Predictors of postconcussive symptoms 3 months after mild traumatic brain injury. Neuropsychology 2012;26(3): 304–13.

140. Clarke LA, Genat RC, Anderson JF. Long-term cognitive complaint and postconcussive symptoms following mild traumatic brain injury: the role of cognitive and affective factors. Brain Inj 2012;26(3):298–307.

141. Yang J, Peek-Asa C, Covassin T, et al. Post-concussion symptoms of depression and anxiety in division I collegiate athletes. Dev Neuropsychol 2015; 40(1):18–23.

142. Silverberg N, Gardner AJ, Brubacher J, et al. Systematic review of multivariable prognostic models for mild traumatic brain injury. J Neurotrauma 2015;32(8): 517–26.
143. Waljas M, Iverson GL, Lange RT, et al. A prospective biopsychosocial study of the persistent post-concussion symptoms following mild traumatic brain injury. J Neurotrauma 2015;32(8):534–47.
144. Wilkins SA, Shannon CN, Brown ST, et al. Establishment of a multidisciplinary concussion program: impact of standardization on patient care and resource utilization. J Neurosurg Pediatr 2014;13(1):82–9.
145. Meehan WP 3rd, d'Hemecourt P, Comstock RD. High school concussions in the 2008-2009 academic year: mechanism, symptoms, and management. Am J Sports Med 2010;38(12):2405–9.
146. Lau B, Lovell MR, Collins MW, et al. Neurocognitive and symptom predictors of recovery in high school athletes. Clin J Sport Med 2009;19(3):216–21.
147. Mihalik JP, Stump JE, Collins MW, et al. Posttraumatic migraine characteristics in athletes following sports-related concussion. J Neurosurg 2005;102(5):850–5.
148. Ventura RE, Jancuska JM, Balcer LJ, et al. Diagnostic tests for concussion: is vision part of the puzzle? J Neuroophthalmol 2015;35(1):73–81.
149. Master CL, Scheiman M, Gallaway M, et al. Vision diagnoses are common after concussion in adolescents. Clin Pediatr (Phila) 2016;55(3):260–7.
150. Heinmiller L, Gunton KB. A review of the current practice in diagnosis and management of visual complaints associated with concussion and postconcussion syndrome. Curr Opin Ophthalmol 2016;27(5):407–12.
151. Rouse MW, Borsting EJ, Mitchell GL, et al. Validity and reliability of the revised convergence insufficiency symptom survey in adults. Ophthalmic Physiol Opt 2004;24(5):384–90.
152. Horan LA, Ticho BH, Khammar AJ, et al. Is the convergence insufficiency symptom survey specific for convergence insufficiency? a prospective, randomized study. Am Orthopt J 2015;65:99–103.
153. Scheiman M, Mitchell GL, Cotter S, et al. A randomized clinical trial of vision therapy/orthoptics versus pencil pushups for the treatment of convergence insufficiency in young adults. Optom Vis Sci 2005;82(7):583–95.
154. Broglio SP, Collins MW, Williams RM, et al. Current and emerging rehabilitation for concussion: a review of the evidence. Clin Sports Med 2015;34(2):213–31.
155. Register-Mihalik JK, Mihalik JP, Guskiewicz KM. Balance deficits after sports-related concussion in individuals reporting posttraumatic headache. Neurosurgery 2008;63(1):76–80 [discussion: 80–2].
156. De Marco AP, Broshek DK. Computerized cognitive testing in the management of youth sports-related concussion. J Child Neurol 2014;31(1):68–75.
157. Broshek DK, De Marco AP, Freeman JR. A review of post-concussion syndrome and psychological factors associated with concussion. Brain Inj 2015;29(2): 228–37.
158. Nelson LD, Tarima S, LaRoche AA, et al. Preinjury somatization symptoms contribute to clinical recovery after sport-related concussion. Neurology 2016; 86(20):1856–63.
159. Mittenberg W, Tremont G, Zielinski RE, et al. Cognitive-behavioral prevention of postconcussion syndrome. Arch Clin Neuropsychol 1996;11(2):139–45.

Exercise in Pregnancy

Vanessa H. Gregg, MD*, James E. Ferguson II, MD, MBA

KEYWORDS

- Exercise - Pregnancy - Maternal outcomes - Fetal outcomes

KEY POINTS

- Regular exercise is recommended for healthy pregnant women.
- Even those who have not been physically active can start a new exercise program gradually during pregnancy.
- Regular exercise during pregnancy promotes overall wellness and helps maintain appropriate gestational weight gain and appropriate fetal weight gain. Exercise in pregnancy may also reduce hypertensive disorders of pregnancy and gestational diabetes, and may be associated with shorter first stage of labor and decreased risk for cesarean section.
- Elite athletes can continue to be highly active, but some modifications may be needed during pregnancy.

INTRODUCTION

Regular exercise confers significant benefits for health and wellness. National guidelines from the US Department of Health and Human Services (HHS) and the American College of Obstetrics and Gynecology (ACOG) advise that all healthy pregnant women should engage routinely in exercise, after consultation with a care provider.[1,2] Exercise is safe and beneficial for most pregnant women and their fetuses, within parameters as described by expert consensus as summarized by the ACOG Committee Opinion and other expert guidance.

EXPERT GUIDELINES AND RECOMMENDATIONS REGARDING EXERCISE DURING PREGNANCY

American College of Sports Medicine Position Stand on Exercise

The American College of Sports Medicine's Position Stand on Exercise points out that regular exercise has numerous benefits for physical and mental health. "The scientific evidence demonstrating the beneficial effects of exercise is indisputable, and the

Conflict of Interest and Financial Disclosure Statements: The authors report no conflict of interest.
Department of Obstetrics and Gynecology, University of Virginia School of Medicine, Charlottesville, VA, USA
* Corresponding author. 2955 Ivy Road, Suite 304, Charlottesville, VA 22903.
E-mail address: Vanessa.Gregg@virginia.edu

benefits of exercise far outweigh the risks in most adults."[3] The American College of Sports Medicine advises continuing an existing exercise program or initiation of a regular exercise program during pregnancy.[4]

US Department of Health and Human Services Physical Activity Guidelines

The 2008 physical activity guidelines from HHS offer specific guidance for exercise in pregnancy:

- "Healthy women who are not already highly active or doing vigorous-intensity aerobic activity should get at least 150 minutes of moderate-intensity aerobic activity per week during pregnancy and the postpartum period. Preferably, this activity should be spread throughout the week."
- "Pregnant women who habitually engage in vigorous-intensity aerobic activity or are highly active can continue physical activity during pregnancy and the postpartum period, provided that they remain healthy and discuss with their health care provider how and when activity should be adjusted over time."

American College of Obstetrics and Gynecology Committee Opinion #650

The ACOG Committee Opinion #650 states that[1]:

- Physical activity in pregnancy has minimal risks and has been shown to benefit most women, although some modification to exercise routines may be necessary because of normal anatomic and physiologic changes and fetal requirements.
- Women with uncomplicated pregnancies should be encouraged to engage in aerobic and strength-conditioning exercises before, during and after pregnancy.

BENEFITS OF EXERCISE DURING PREGNANCY

There are numerous health benefits associated with exercise during pregnancy. The available literature is variable in what it explores and the strength of the findings. This article reviews the current available evidence regarding exercise and the maintenance of healthy weight gain, decreasing gestational hypertension, reducing maternal back pain during pregnancy, shortening the duration of labor, and reducing the risk for cesarean section.

Improve or Maintain Fitness

A 2006 Cochrane Review (updated 2010) evaluated 14 controlled trials of exercise in pregnancy. Pregnant women who exercised at least two to three times per week seemed to improve or maintain their fitness level. There was not sufficient data to draw more specific conclusions about maternal and infant benefits or risks.[5]

A more recent small, randomized trial of sedentary pregnant women evaluated a supervised aerobic training program involving 45- to 60-minute exercise activities at moderate intensity, 4 days per week. Results showed increased aerobic fitness and strength in the exercise group compared with control subjects, with no significant difference in pregnancy outcomes.[6]

Maintain Healthy Weight Gain

A 2006 Cochrane Review (updated 2015) evaluated randomized controlled trials of diet and exercise interventions and their effects on gestational weight gain. Women who received exercise interventions were more likely to have low gestational weight gain than control subjects.[7] A meta-analysis of randomized trials of structured exercise programs in pregnancy showed similar findings of reduced maternal weight gain with structured exercise programs.[8]

Decrease Gestational Hypertension

A 2006 review of studies evaluating prescribed moderate-intensity aerobic exercise compared with maintenance of normal activity during pregnancy found no significant difference in the development of preeclampsia between the exercise group and the nonexercising group.[9] A Cochrane review of diet and exercise interventions during pregnancy found no difference in the development of preeclampsia when comparing women who exercised with those who did not. However, in that review, women who participated in an exercise program during pregnancy were less likely to have hypertension during pregnancy.[7]

Another dose-response meta-analysis of observational studies evaluating physical activity and risk of preeclampsia found that increasing levels of physical activity before and during pregnancy were inversely associated with the development of preeclampsia. The more women exercised before and during their pregnancies, the less likely they were to develop preeclampsia.[10] There is mixed-quality evidence from which to draw conclusions, but there is a possible association between exercising and a decreased risk of hypertensive disorders of pregnancy.

Reduce Back Pain

A survey of 950 pregnant women (84% response rate) showed that low back pain is a common complaint in pregnancy, with 68.5% of respondents reporting low back pain during their pregnancies.[11] A review of randomized controlled trials of interventions to reduce back pain in pregnancy found that any land-based exercise was associated with a significant reduction in back pain and improvement in functional disability.[12]

Shorten Labor

A recent randomized controlled trial conducted in Spain evaluated a prescribed physical conditioning program and its effects on outcomes. The investigators found a significant reduction in the first stage of labor among women who followed a prescribed exercise program compared with the control group.[13]

Reduce Risk of Cesarean Section

Women who participated in structured physical exercise programs were less likely to require cesarean delivery than women who did not participate in such programs.[1,6,8,14]

MATERNAL PHYSIOLOGY OF PREGNANCY

It is clear that exercise during pregnancy is associated with numerous salutary outcomes. However, before exercise is prescribed, it is important that providers understand physiologic changes associated with pregnancy, and those associated with exercise in pregnancy.

Cardiovascular and Pulmonary Adaptations

There are many physiologic changes that occur during pregnancy. There are significant cardiovascular changes, including a significant increase in blood volume, heart rate, and cardiac output, and a decrease in systemic vascular resistance. In healthy pregnancies, blood pressure decreases, beginning in early pregnancy, with a nadir in mid-pregnancy. Heart rate and blood pressure typically normalize quickly in the postpartum period in the absence of superimposed complications.[15] Pulmonary changes include increased oxygen consumption and minute ventilation, and decreased functional residual capacity and oxygen reserve.[16,17] **Table 1** summarizes the cardiovascular and pulmonary adaptations that occur during normal pregnancy.

Glucose Metabolism

Maternal physiologic changes in carbohydrate metabolism during pregnancy serve to ensure a constant supply of glucose to the fetus to sustain growth. Glucose crosses the placenta to the fetus by means of facilitated diffusion, a process by which the glucose is diffused across cell membranes by carrier proteins. Consequently in the fasting state maternal fasting glucose levels are decreased by 15% to 20% compared with those in nonpregnant women.[19] The lowered glucose levels are associated with decreases in plasma insulin, producing an "accelerated and exaggerated response to starvation."[19] Feeding produces hyperglycemia, an increase in serum insulin levels, and hypertriglyceridemia. There is also a diminished response to insulin caused by human placental lactogen and other hormones.

Musculoskeletal Changes

There are multiple physiologic changes in pregnancy that impact the musculoskeletal system. There is a variable increase in body mass, and the distribution of body mass changes with the growth of the uterus and fetus.[20] Relaxation of the peripheral joints is a normal physiologic process in pregnancy and has been confirmed in multiple studies, leading to increased joint laxity.[21] There is usually progressive lordosis and a change in the center of gravity.[22]

A three-dimensional gait analysis of 15 pregnant women in the third trimester of pregnancy showed alteration in several kinetic parameters, including increased use of hip abductor, hip extensor, and ankle plantar flexor muscle groups. These alterations are likely adaptive to compensate for the physiologic changes in the center of gravity and the increased lordosis of pregnancy.[20]

Weight Gain in Pregnancy

The Institute of Medicine (IOM) has published and revised guidelines for recommended weight gain in pregnancy, which varies based on the prepregnancy body mass index. The IOM recommendations are summarized in **Table 2**. The goal of the guidelines is to define appropriate weight gain to promote normal infant birth weight, and to reduce postpartum weight retention.[23]

A systematic literature review of birth outcomes associated with gestational weight gain confirmed that there was an association between appropriate gestational weight

Table 1
Cardiovascular and pulmonary adaptations in pregnancy

Cardiovascular		Pulmonary	
Blood volume	Increased, can be 40%–45%	Oxygen consumption	Increased, 10%–20% at rest
Heart rate	Increased 10 bpm	Minute ventilation	Increased 40%–50%
Cardiac output	Increased	Functional residual capacity	Decreased
Systemic vascular resistance	Decreased systemic vascular resistance	Oxygen reserve	Decreased

Data from Refs.[15–18]

Table 2		
Institute of Medicine's recommended weight gain based on body mass index		
Prepregnancy Weight	**Body Mass Index**	**Recommended Weight Gain (lb)**
Underweight	<18.5	28–40
Normal weight	18.5–24.9	25–35
Overweight	25–29.9	15–25
Obese	≥30	11–20

Data from Institute of Medicine, I.O.M.P.W.G. National Research Council Committee to Reexamine. 2009; and American College of Obstetricians and Gynecologists. ACOG committee opinion No. 548: weight gain during pregnancy. Obstet Gynecol 2013;121(1):210–2.

gain as defined by the IOM and the outcomes of having a normal-range birthweight baby with normal fetal growth. In addition, the same review found that gestational weight gain within the IOM guidelines was associated with less postpartum weight retention. This review further identified that there was strong evidence that excess gestational weight gain was associated with increased infant birthweight, whereas insufficient weight gain was associated with lower infant birth weight.[24]

PHYSIOLOGIC CHANGES ASSOCIATED WITH EXERCISE DURING PREGNANCY
Maternal Cardiovascular Physiology Changes with Exercise

Research suggests that exercise performed during pregnancy can improve cardiovascular function in pregnant women without compromising fetal well-being.[5,25–27] Heart rate variability is a measure of cardiac autonomic nervous system function, which is a measure of cardiovascular health. A recent study of healthy pregnant women assessed heart rate variability with exercise in pregnancy. The results showed that consistent maternal exercise throughout pregnancy was associated with lower maternal heart rate and increased heart rate variability, suggesting overall improved cardiac autonomic control.[28]

Maternal Glucose Metabolism During Exercise

A study of glucose metabolism in pregnancy evaluated glucose homeostasis in the third trimester in response to exercise, compared with glucose homeostasis in a nonpregnant control group. Results showed that pregnant women had more rapid and extreme drops in blood glucose with exercise compared with nonpregnant control subjects. In addition, pregnant women had more significantly decreased insulin levels after exercise.[29]

Fetal Physiology During Exercise

Just as maternal physiology is affected by exercise, so is fetal physiology. The fetal heart rate has been shown to increase as a result of maternal exercise, both during and soon after the exercise occurs.[1,18,30] A research study evaluated exercise treadmill tests in pregnant women of varying fitness levels, with exercise intensities that were appropriate to the prepregnancy activity levels of the participants, based on HHS guidelines. Assessments of fetal well-being were made before and after the treadmill exercise sessions. The results indicated that maternal treadmill exercise was well-tolerated by the fetuses in this study.[31] These results confirm that light-to-moderate-intensity exercise during pregnancy is well-tolerated by the fetus.

EXERCISE PRESCRIPTION

Pregnant women are often more receptive than their nonpregnant counterparts to life-style modification and health counseling. Exercise is encouraged for pregnant women; however, physicians must evaluate each individual pregnant woman before prescribing her optimal exercise regimen.

The HHS guidelines recommend that pregnant women should work with their care providers to tailor their exercise programs appropriately based on their prepregnancy fitness levels and any complications in the pregnancies. Women who are starting a new exercise program should increase their physical activity gradually over time.[2]

The ACOG Committee Opinion recommends that the pregnant patient should have a medical evaluation to ensure that it is safe for her to pursue an exercise program during her pregnancy. ACOG provides specific guidance regarding activities to encourage, and those to avoid, during pregnancy. In a prior guideline, ACOG had recommended limiting the maximum heart rate to 140 beats per minute during exercise in pregnancy. However, that limitation is no longer included in the updated guideline, published in 2015. Rather, ACOG now recommends the use of perceived exertion as a self-guide to limiting exertion during exercise.[1,32,33]

It must be remembered that prescriptions for exercise during pregnancy may impact two individuals and thus maternal and fetal well-being must be considered.

Recommended Exercise Types: American College of Obstetrics and Gynecology Committee Opinion

ACOG has provided specific guidance on exercise activities that are considered safe in pregnancy. These activities are recommended for healthy women who are cleared for exercise in pregnancy. Walking, swimming, stationery cycling, and low-impact aerobics are all preferred forms of exercise in pregnancy. Yoga and pilates are considered safe, if care is taken to avoid positions that could cause hypotension. Running, jogging, and strength-training are considered safe but should be discussed first with an obstetric care provider. Racquet sports may be acceptable, although activities with an increased risk of abrupt loss of balance and falls should be avoided.[1]

Exercises to Avoid in Pregnancy: American College of Obstetrics and Gynecology Committee Opinion

Contact sports should be avoided because of the risk of trauma. In addition, activities with a significant risk of falls or trauma should be avoided, including skiing, water skiing, surfing, off-road cycling, horseback riding, and gymnastics. Scuba diving, sky diving and hot yoga are not recommended in pregnancy.[1] **Box 1** summarizes the relative contraindications to aerobic exercise in pregnancy, as recommended by ACOG, and **Box 2** summarizes the absolute contraindications. Individual recommendations should be made with the advice of an obstetric care provider.

LIMITATIONS AND CONTRAINDICATIONS TO EXERCISE DURING PREGNANCY

Pregnant women should be careful to maintain adequate nutrition and hydration with exercise.[1,29] Although it is unlikely that body core temperatures would exceed 39°C, the Royal College of Obstetricians and Gynaecologists recommends limiting exposure during exercise to temperatures exceeding 90°F and keeping hydrotherapy pool temperatures less than or equal to 95°F.[34] Because of anatomic and physiologic changes associated with pregnancy, there is increased risk of hypotension with exercise. In particular, activities that require flat supine positioning can increase

Box 1
Relative contraindications to aerobic exercise during pregnancy

- Anemia
- Unevaluated maternal cardiac arrhythmia
- Chronic bronchitis
- Poorly controlled type 1 diabetes
- Extreme morbid obesity
- Extreme underweight (body mass index <12)
- History of extremely sedentary lifestyle
- Intrauterine growth restriction in current pregnancy
- Poorly controlled hypertension
- Orthopedic limitations
- Poorly controlled seizure disorder
- Poorly controlled hyperthyroidism
- Heavy smoker

this risk, and therefore should be avoided. Increased musculoskeletal discomforts or injuries could be a complication of exercise in pregnancy because of increased laxity and altered center of gravity, and care should be taken to avoid activities that increase the risk of musculoskeletal injuries.[6,20,35] ACOG provides specific warning signs for discontinuation of exercise during pregnancy, as summarized in **Box 3**.

FETAL OUTCOMES WITH MATERNAL EXERCISE DURING PREGNANCY

Pregnant women can be reassured that maternal exercise in pregnancy is generally well-tolerated by the fetus.[1,31]

Box 2
Absolute contraindications to aerobic exercise during pregnancy

- Hemodynamically significant heart disease
- Restrictive lung disease
- Incompetent cervix or cerclage
- Multiple gestation at risk of premature labor
- Persistent second- or third-trimester bleeding
- Placenta previa after 26 weeks of gestation
- Premature labor during the current pregnancy
- Ruptured membranes
- Preeclampsia or pregnancy-induced hypertension
- Severe anemia

Box 3
Warning signs to discontinue exercise while pregnant

- Vaginal bleeding
- Regular painful contractions
- Amniotic fluid leakage
- Dyspnea before exertion
- Dizziness
- Headache
- Chest pain
- Muscle weakness affecting balance
- Calf pain or swelling

Effects of Maternal Exercise on Fetal Growth and Birthweight

Some studies have suggested that exercise during pregnancy does not significantly alter birthweight. A meta-analysis found that mean birthweight for infants born to mothers who exercised was similar to those born to control, nonexercising mothers. However, the researchers found that women who continued vigorous exercise in the third trimester delivered infants who weighed 200 to 400 g less than the infants of their nonexercising counterparts.[36]

A more recent meta-analysis reviewed randomized controlled trials in pregnant women comparing a supervised exercise intervention with a group receiving usual prenatal care. In this group of 36 trials, pregnant women who exercised were less likely to have a large-for-gestational-age newborn, with no change in the likelihood of having a small-for-gestational-age newborn. In this study, mean weight gain in pregnancy was less among those who participated in the exercise protocol than among those who did not.[37] Thus, the best evidence available suggests that prescribed moderate-intensity exercise during pregnancy does not adversely affect infant weight at birth.

Maternal Exercise and Preterm Birth

A recent meta-analysis of randomized clinical trials of exercise programs during pregnancy evaluated studies of aerobic exercise for 35 to 90 minutes, performed three to four times weekly, found that there was no significant difference in the rate of preterm birth for women who exercised compared with those who did not. The mean gestational age at delivery was similar among those prescribed an exercise program and those who were not. There were no significant differences in low birthweight babies or in mean infant weight at delivery.[38] This analysis confirms that among sedentary women with a normal, singleton pregnancy, moderate-intensity exercise does not seem to increase the risk of preterm birth or earlier delivery. This review also confirmed previous findings that moderate-intensity exercise does not adversely affect infant birthweight.

A recent Norwegian study evaluated 188 children whose mothers had participated in a structured exercise program during their pregnancies compared with a control group whose mothers had not participated in an exercise program during their pregnancies. Assessments of cognitive, language, and motor skills were undertaken at 18 months of age. Results indicated that there were no adverse neurodevelopmental effects on the children whose mothers had participated in exercise during pregnancy.[39]

OTHER CONSIDERATIONS
High Performance Exercise During Pregnancy

Serena Williams, a professional tennis athlete, recently won the Australian Open professional tennis tournament during her first trimester of pregnancy, garnering a great deal of public interest. The HHS and ACOG guidelines for exercise in pregnancy state that it is safe and reasonable for pregnant women who are already participating in vigorous-intensity aerobic activity to continue to be highly active during pregnancy, in conjunction with advice from their care providers.[1,2]

Pregnant elite athletes need provider supervision to ensure safe progression of exercise during pregnancy. Physiologic changes associated with pregnancy may necessitate alteration in training routines. High-performing athletes may need additional nutritional support to ensure adequate pregnancy weight gain.[40]

Providing advice to elite athletes during pregnancy is challenging for providers because there is no uniform agreement on what defines an "elite athlete." Moreover, it is difficult in practical terms to define and measure degree of exertion during exercise, and there are few studies (typically only with small numbers of patients) on which to draw conclusions when advising patients. A reasonable definition is an athlete who trains year round at a high level. Training is likely to be at least 5 days per week, averaging close to 2 hours per day and meet or exceed 6 metabolic equivalents level used to describe vigorous physical activity.[41]

In a study of high-performing pregnant athletes, six Olympic-level pregnant women were studied at 23 to 29 weeks of gestation on a treadmill exercise activity at approximately 60% to 90% of maximal oxygen consumption. Fetal heart rate was within the normal range as long as the mother exercised less than 90% of maximal maternal heart rate. In some instances when maternal heart rate exceeded 90% of maximal, there was a simultaneous reduction in uterine volume blood flow to less than 50% of the initial value and fetal heart rate decelerations. Overall, however, all fetuses did well. It was concluded that exercise at less than 90% of maximal maternal heart rate may be regarded as a safety zone for elite athletes.[42]

In a subsequent similar study, it was likewise found that the fetuses of a subset of highly active pregnant women (whose conditioning was less than that of an elite athlete) had transient heart rate decelerations following strenuous exercise. These changes were often accompanied by increased resistance in the umbilical and uterine artery Doppler parameters and did not occur when the maternal heart rate was less than or equal to 84% of maximal.[31,32] Although the clinical significance of the transient fetal decelerations and increased vascular impedance is unknown, a conservative course might target strenuous exercise in pregnancy to achieve maternal heart rates less than or equal to 84% of maximum.

Specific counseling to elite athletes regarding exercise during pregnancy should include advice regarding limitations to maximum exertion, precautions to minimize risk of injury, and vigilance for potential indicators of overexertion. **Table 3** provides examples of specific guidelines for elite athletes regarding exercise during pregnancy.

Postpartum Exercise

Regular exercise during pregnancy can help to achieve recommended gestational weight gain. Adherence to recommended guidelines for weight gain in pregnancy can help to reduce postpartum weight retention.[24] Investigators have observed that women tend to have decreased exercise participation after giving birth, and sedentary lifestyles for these women can contribute to the development of obesity and

Table 3
Risks of exercise in pregnancy for the elite athlete

Risks	Guidelines
Maternal	
Musculoskeletal injuries	With evidence of joint and ligament laxity, individualize and modify training
Cardiovascular complications	Be vigilant of warning signs, including palpitations and tachycardia at rest or any signs of orthostatic hypotension
Threatened abortion or premature labor	Stop training
Hypoglycemia	Prevent hypoglycemia by following proper nutritional guidelines
Fetal	
Fetal distress	Be alert to fetal movements or activity; in the presence of any complication, stop training and resume only after medical clearance
Intrauterine growth restriction	Stop training
Fetal malformations	Avoid hyperthermia and dehydration immediately after conception and for weeks thereafter
Fetal injuries	Avoid sports with a high probability of blunt trauma after 16–20 wk of gestation

Reprinted from Artal R, Hopkins S. Clinical updates in women's health care: exercise. Vol. XII, No. 2, 2013; with permission from ACOG.

associated metabolic disorders.[43,44] Regular exercise should be encouraged in the postpartum period, as soon as it is deemed medically safe to participate in such exercise.[1]

REFERENCES

1. ACOG committee opinion No. 650: physical activity and exercise during pregnancy and the postpartum period. Obstet Gynecol 2015;126(6):e135–42.
2. US Department of Health and Human Services. Physical activity guidelines advisory committee report 2008:A1-H14. Washington, DC: U.S. Department of Health and Human Services; 2008.
3. Garber CE, Blissmer B, Deschenes MR, et al. American College of Sports Medicine position stand. Quantity and quality of exercise for developing and maintaining cardiorespiratory, musculoskeletal, and neuromotor fitness in apparently healthy adults: guidance for prescribing exercise. Med Sci Sports Exerc 2011; 43(7):1334–59.
4. American College of Sports Medicine. ACSM's guidelines for exercise testing and prescription. In: American College of Sports Medicine, editor. ACSM's guidelines for exercise testing and prescription. 9th edition. Philadelphia: Wolters Kluwer/ Lippincott Williams & Wilkins Health; 2014.
5. Kramer MS, McDonald SW. Aerobic exercise for women during pregnancy. Cochrane Database Syst Rev 2006;(3):CD000180.
6. Price BB, Amini SB, Kappeler K. Exercise in pregnancy: effect on fitness and obstetric outcomes. A randomized trial. Med Sci Sports Exerc 2012;44(12):2263–9.

7. Muktabhant B, Lawrie TA, Lumbiganon P, et al. Diet or exercise, or both, for preventing excessive weight gain in pregnancy. Cochrane Database Syst Rev 2015;(6):CD007145.

8. Domenjoz I, Kayser B, Boulvain M. Effect of physical activity during pregnancy on mode of delivery. Am J Obstet Gynecol 2014;211(4):401.e1-11.

9. Meher S, Duley L. Exercise or other physical activity for preventing pre-eclampsia and its complications. Cochrane Database Syst Rev 2006;(2):CD005942.

10. Aune D, Saugstad OD, Henriksen T, et al. Physical activity and the risk of preeclampsia: a systematic review and meta-analysis. Epidemiology 2014;25(3):331–43.

11. Wang SM, Dezinno P, Maranets I, et al. Low back pain during pregnancy: prevalence, risk factors, and outcomes. Obstet Gynecol 2004;104(1):65–70.

12. Liddle SD, Pennick V. Interventions for preventing and treating low-back and pelvic pain during pregnancy. Cochrane Database Syst Rev 2015;(9):CD001139.

13. Perales M, Santos-Lozano A, Ruiz JR, et al. Benefits of aerobic or resistance training during pregnancy on maternal health and perinatal outcomes: a systematic review. Early Hum Dev 2016;94:43–8.

14. Barakat R, Pelaez M, Lopez C, et al. Exercise during pregnancy reduces the rate of cesarean and instrumental deliveries: results of a randomized controlled trial. J Matern Fetal Neonatal Med 2012;25(11):2372–6.

15. Mahendru AA, Everett TR, Wilkinson IB, et al. Maternal cardiovascular changes from pre-pregnancy to very early pregnancy. J Hypertens 2012;30(11):2168–72.

16. Artal R, Wiswell R, Romem Y, et al. Pulmonary responses to exercise in pregnancy. Am J Obstet Gynecol 1986;154(2):378–83.

17. Hegewald MJ, Crapo RO. Respiratory physiology in pregnancy. Clin Chest Med 2011;32(1):1–13, vii.

18. Artal R, Rutherford S, Romem Y, et al. Fetal heart rate responses to maternal exercise. Am J Obstet Gynecol 1986;155(4):729–33.

19. Barclay M. Physiology of pregnancy. Global Library of Women's Medicine 2009. Available at: http://www.glowm.com/section_view/item/103#16901. Accessed March 14, 2017.

20. Foti T, Davids JR, Bagley A. A biomechanical analysis of gait during pregnancy. J Bone Joint Surg Am 2000;82(5):625–32.

21. Marnach ML, Ramin KD, Ramsey PS, et al. Characterization of the relationship between joint laxity and maternal hormones in pregnancy. Obstet Gynecol 2003;101(2):331–5.

22. Williams Obstetrics LK, Cunningham F, Bloom SL, et al, editors. Maternal physiology. New York: McGraw-Hill; 2013.

23. Institute of Medicine. Weight gain during pregnancy: reexamining the guidelines. Washington, DC: National Academies Press; 2009.

24. Siega-Riz AM, Viswanathan M, Moos MK, et al. A systematic review of outcomes of maternal weight gain according to the Institute of Medicine recommendations: birthweight, fetal growth, and postpartum weight retention. Am J Obstet Gynecol 2009;201(4):339.e1-14.

25. Prather H, Spitznagle T, Hunt D. Benefits of exercise during pregnancy. PM R 2012;4(11):845–50 [quiz: 850].

26. Kalisiak B, Spitznagle T. What effect does an exercise program for healthy pregnant women have on the mother, fetus, and child? PM R 2009;1(3):261–6.

27. Davies GA, Wolfe LA, Mottola MF, et al. Joint SOGC/CSEP clinical practice guideline: exercise in pregnancy and the postpartum period. Can J Appl Physiol 2003;28(3):330–41.

28. May LE, Knowlton J, Hanson J, et al. Effects of exercise during pregnancy on maternal heart rate and heart rate variability. PM R 2016;8(7):611–7.
29. Soultanakis HN, Artal R, Wiswell RA. Prolonged exercise in pregnancy: glucose homeostasis, ventilatory and cardiovascular responses. Semin Perinatol 1996; 20(4):315–27.
30. Carpenter MW, Sady SP, Hoegsberg B, et al. Fetal heart rate response to maternal exertion. JAMA 1988;259(20):3006–9.
31. Szymanski LM, Satin AJ. Exercise during pregnancy: fetal responses to current public health guidelines. Obstet Gynecol 2012;119(3):603–10.
32. Szymanski LM, Satin AJ. Strenuous exercise during pregnancy: is there a limit? Am J Obstet Gynecol 2012;207(3):179.e1-6.
33. American College of Obstetrics and Gynecology. Exercise during pregnancy and the postpartum period. ACOG technical bulletin No. 189–February 1994. Int J Gynaecol Obstet 1994;45:65–70.
34. Royal College of Obstetricians and Gynecologists. Exercise in pregnancy. 2006. Available at: http://www.nice.org.uk. Accessed March 10, 2017.
35. Impact of physical activity during pregnancy and postpartum on chronic disease risk. Med Sci Sports Exerc 2006;38(5):989–1006.
36. Leet T, Flick L. Effect of exercise on birthweight. Clin Obstet Gynecol 2003;46(2): 423–31.
37. Wiebe HW, Boulé NG, Chari R, et al. The effect of supervised prenatal exercise on fetal growth: a meta-analysis. Obstet Gynecol 2015;125(5):1185–94.
38. Di Mascio D, Magro-Malosso ER, Saccone G, et al. Exercise during pregnancy in normal-weight women and risk of preterm birth: a systematic review and meta-analysis of randomized controlled trials. Am J Obstet Gynecol 2016;215(5): 561–71.
39. Hellenes OM, Vik T, Løhaugen GC, et al. Regular moderate exercise during pregnancy does not have an adverse effect on the neurodevelopment of the child. Acta Paediatr 2015;104(3):285–91.
40. Artal R, Hopkins S. Exercise. Clin Update Womens Health Care 2013;12:1.
41. Pivarnik JM, Szymanski LM, Conway MR. The elite athlete and strenuous exercise in pregnancy. Clin Obstet Gynecol 2016;59(3):613–9.
42. Salvesen KA, Hem E, Sundgot-Borgen J. Fetal wellbeing may be compromised during strenuous exercise among pregnant elite athletes. Br J Sports Med 2012;46(4):279–83.
43. Minig L, Trimble EL, Sarsotti C, et al. Building the evidence base for postoperative and postpartum advice. Obstet Gynecol 2009;114(4):892–900.
44. O'Toole ML, Sawicki MA, Artal R. Structured diet and physical activity prevent postpartum weight retention. J Womens Health (Larchmt) 2003;12(10):991–8.

UNITED STATES POSTAL SERVICE® Statement of Ownership, Management, and Circulation
(All Periodicals Publications Except Requester Publications)

1. Publication Title	2. Publication Number		3. Filing Date
CLINICS IN SPORTS MEDICINE	0 0 0 – 7 0 2		9/18/2017

4. Issue Frequency	5. Number of Issues Published Annually	6. Annual Subscription Price
JAN, APR, JUL, OCT	4	$343.00

7. Complete Mailing Address of Known Office of Publication (Not printer) (Street, city, county, state, and ZIP+4®)

ELSEVIER INC.
230 Park Avenue, Suite 800
New York, NY 10169

Contact Person
STEPHEN R. BUSHING

Telephone (Include area code)
215-239-3688

8. Complete Mailing Address of Headquarters or General Business Office of Publisher (Not printer)

ELSEVIER INC.
230 Park Avenue, Suite 800
New York, NY 10169

9. Full Names and Complete Mailing Addresses of Publisher, Editor, and Managing Editor (Do not leave blank)

Publisher (Name and complete mailing address)

ADRIANNE BRIGIDO, ELSEVIER INC.
1600 JOHN F KENNEDY BLVD. SUITE 1800
PHILADELPHIA, PA 19103-2899

Editor (Name and complete mailing address)

LAUREN BOYLE, ELSEVIER INC.
1600 JOHN F KENNEDY BLVD. SUITE 1800
PHILADELPHIA, PA 19103-2899

Managing Editor (Name and complete mailing address)

PATRICK MANLEY, ELSEVIER INC.
1600 JOHN F KENNEDY BLVD. SUITE 1800
PHILADELPHIA, PA 19103-2899

10. Owner (Do not leave blank. If the publication is owned by a corporation, give the name and address of the corporation immediately followed by the names and addresses of all stockholders owning or holding 1 percent or more of the total amount of stock. If not owned by a corporation, give the names and addresses of the individual owners. If owned by a partnership or other unincorporated firm, give its name and address as well as those of each individual owner. If the publication is published by a nonprofit organization, give its name and address.)

Full Name	Complete Mailing Address
WHOLLY OWNED SUBSIDIARY OF REED/ELSEVIER, US HOLDINGS	1600 JOHN F KENNEDY BLVD. SUITE 1800 PHILADELPHIA, PA 19103-2899

11. Known Bondholders, Mortgagees, and Other Security Holders Owning or Holding 1 Percent or More of Total Amount of Bonds, Mortgages, or Other Securities. If none, check box ► ☐ None

Full Name	Complete Mailing Address
N/A	

12. Tax Status (For completion by nonprofit organizations authorized to mail at nonprofit rates) (Check one)
The purpose, function, and nonprofit status of this organization and the exempt status for federal income tax purposes:
☒ Has Not Changed During Preceding 12 Months
☐ Has Changed During Preceding 12 Months (Publisher must submit explanation of change with this statement)

13. Publication Title	14. Issue Date for Circulation Data Below
CLINICS IN SPORTS MEDICINE	JULY 2017

15. Extent and Nature of Circulation		Average No. Copies Each Issue During Preceding 12 Months	No. Copies of Single Issue Published Nearest to Filing Date
a. Total Number of Copies (Net press run)		382	299
b. Paid Circulation (By Mail and Outside the Mail)	(1) Mailed Outside-County Paid Subscriptions Stated on PS Form 3541 (Include paid distribution above nominal rate, advertiser's proof copies, and exchange copies)	193	178
	(2) Mailed In-County Paid Subscriptions Stated on PS Form 3541 (Include paid distribution above nominal rate, advertiser's proof copies, and exchange copies)	0	0
	(3) Paid Distribution Outside the Mails Including Sales Through Dealers and Carriers, Street Vendors, Counter Sales, and Other Paid Distribution Outside USPS®	50	50
	(4) Paid Distribution by Other Classes of Mail Through the USPS (e.g. First-Class Mail®)	0	0
c. Total Paid Distribution (Sum of 15b (1), (2), (3), and (4))	►	243	228
d. Free or Nominal Rate Distribution (By Mail and Outside the Mail)	(1) Free or Nominal Rate Outside-County Copies included on PS Form 3541	71	71
	(2) Free or Nominal Rate In-County Copies Included on PS Form 3541	0	0
	(3) Free or Nominal Rate Copies Mailed at Other Classes Through the USPS (e.g. First-Class Mail)	0	0
	(4) Free or Nominal Rate Distribution Outside the Mail (Carriers or other means)	0	0
e. Total Free or Nominal Rate Distribution (Sum of 15d (1), (2), (3) and (4))	►	71	71
f. Total Distribution (Sum of 15c and 15e)	►	314	299
g. Copies not Distributed (See Instructions to Publishers #4 (page #3))	►	68	0
h. Total (Sum of 15f and g)	►	382	299
i. Percent Paid (15c divided by 15f times 100)	►	77.39%	76.25%

* If you are claiming electronic copies, go to line 16 on page 3. If you are not claiming electronic copies, skip to line 17 on page 3.

16. Electronic Copy Circulation		Average No. Copies Each Issue During Preceding 12 Months	No. Copies of Single Issue Published Nearest to Filing Date
a. Paid Electronic Copies	►	0	0
b. Total Paid Print Copies (Line 15c) + Paid Electronic Copies (Line 16a)	►	243	228
c. Total Print Distribution (Line 15f) + Paid Electronic Copies (Line 16a)	►	314	299
d. Percent Paid (Both Print & Electronic Copies) (16b divided by 16c × 100)	►	77.39%	76.25%

☒ I certify that 50% of all my distributed copies (electronic and print) are paid above a nominal price.

17. Publication of Statement of Ownership

☒ If the publication is a general publication, publication of this statement is required. Will be printed   ☐ Publication not required

in the OCTOBER 2017 issue of this publication.

18. Signature and Title of Editor, Publisher, Business Manager, or Owner   Date

Stephen R. Bushing   9/18/2017

STEPHEN R. BUSHING - INVENTORY DISTRIBUTION CONTROL MANAGER

I certify that all information furnished on this form is true and complete. I understand that anyone who furnishes false or misleading information on this form or who omits material or information requested on the form may be subject to criminal sanctions (including fines and imprisonment) and/or civil sanctions (including civil penalties).

PS Form **3526**, July 2014 (Page 1 of 4 (see instructions page 4))   PSN: 7530-01-000-9931   PRIVACY NOTICE: See our privacy policy on www.usps.com.

PS Form **3526**, July 2014 (Page 3 of 4)

Moving?

Make sure your subscription moves with you!

To notify us of your new address, find your **Clinics Account Number** (located on your mailing label above your name), and contact customer service at:

Email: journalscustomerservice-usa@elsevier.com

800-654-2452 (subscribers in the U.S. & Canada)
314-447-8871 (subscribers outside of the U.S. & Canada)

Fax number: 314-447-8029

Elsevier Health Sciences Division
Subscription Customer Service
3251 Riverport Lane
Maryland Heights, MO 63043

*To ensure uninterrupted delivery of your subscription,
please notify us at least 4 weeks in advance of move.

Printed and bound by CPI Group (UK) Ltd, Croydon, CR0 4YY

08/05/2025

01864703-0008